THE NURSE MANAGER'S ANSWER BOOK

RUTH I. HANSTEN, RN, MBA
Principal
Hansten & Washburn
Bainbridge Island, Washington

MARILYNN J. WASHBURN, RN, MA
Principal
Hansten & Washburn
Bainbridge Island, Washington

AN ASPEN PUBLICATION®

Aspen Publishers, Inc.
Gaithersburg, Maryland
1994

RT
89
.H37
1994
c.1

Library of Congress Cataloging-in-Publication Data

Hansten, Ruth I.
The nurse manager's answer book /
Ruth I. Hansten, Marilynn J. Washburn.
p.   cm.
Includes bibliographical references and index.
ISBN 0-8342-0501-7
1. Nursing services—Administration. I. Washburn, Marilynn. II. Title.
[DNLM: 1. Nurse Administrators. 2. Nursing organization &
administration. WY 105 H251n 1993]
RT89.H37   1993
362.1'73'068—dc20
DNLM/DLC
for Library of Congress
93-4978
CIP

Z8221938

Copyright © 1994 by Aspen Publishers, Inc.

Aspen Publishers, Inc., grants permission for photocopying for
limited personal or internal use. This consent does not extend to
other kinds of copying, such as copying for general distribu-
tion, for advertising or promotional purposes, for creating new
collective works, or for resale. For information, address Aspen
Publishers, Inc., Permissions Department, 200 Orchard Ridge
Drive, Suite 200, Gaithersburg, Maryland 20878.

Editorial Resources: Lenda Hill
Ruth Bloom

Library of Congress Catalog Card Number: 93-4978
ISBN: 0-8342-0501-7

Printed in the United States of America

1 2 3 4 5

To Marilynn's husband Al, who provided emotional (and computer) support even though he wasn't willing to read the software manual for us, and to her sons Zach, who always offered a hand (if there was money to be made), and Jon, who kept a steady supply of M&Ms handy to make it through the long sessions in the office, and without whose proud boasting to their friends Mom would not have been as inspired (or driven!), and to the laptop computer, which should be at the bottom of the ocean for all the challenges it sent our way!

To Ruth's husband Phil, whose encouragement and belief (and only decaf espresso!) kept us going at the computer late at night; her sons Matt and Kirk, who didn't complain about microwave dinners and have always expected Mom's books to be a success, and without whose impending college bills we may not have been driven to succeed. Ruth also thanks her stepsons Marty and Chris for their comic relief, and especially her stepdaughter Michelle for her ability to sustain Ruth during relief expeditions to the shopping mall while talking about our men! To Periscope (Pudder) for sitting and chewing the manuscript repeatedly as we worked on it.

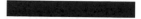

Table of Contents

Foreword

IN THESE TIMES of predictable uncertainty, nurse managers are encircled by the problems of the past—magnified; and by the the new problems of the 1990s: quality; productivity; cost containment; and reform . . . reform . . . reform . . . .

The practical, problem-solving approach of *The Nurse Manager's Answer Book* is easy to access and fun to peruse. A sense of humor combined with a sense of balance and an ability to keep everything in perspective are the essential ingredients for success in this role. This book will give you these ingredients and the formula that helps "the medicine go down."

To paraphrase the president of American Express, this is not the time for predicting rain—rather, we must build the ark. Just do it!

VENNER M. FARLEY, RN, EdD

Dean, Department of Health Professions
Golden West College

President/Principal
Innovative Nursing Consultants (INC)
6512 Kings Crown Road
Orange, California

Foreword

AS WE NEAR the 21st century it is clear that nursing as we know it will not look and feel the same. Change is and will continue to be an everyday occurrence and the reformed health care system will offer new and unfamiliar challenges. Nurses will be expected to provide care to a changing client base using a variety of delivery methods and fewer resources.

Thriving in such an environment will require management skills far beyond those expected in the past. It will be nurses' management expertise and their ability to demonstrate leadership that will ensure the first-class health care delivery the public expects and deserves. Even more critical are the skills nurses will need not only to manage change but to further the results of change. These skills will allow nurses to build a system that has quality service and caring as its outcomes.

Those of us in health care have come to accept the reality that the one constant we will experience, at least for the next several years, is change. Nurses need resources—resources that will help build the repertoire of skills necessary to achieve the best outcomes. *The Nurse Manager's Answer Book* is such a resource. Hansten and Washburn have provided an easy-to-read set of substantive yet handy tips that provide both experienced and new managers with ideas on how to manage better in the current and future health care environments.

From teamwork to handling difficult people to communicating with the JCAHO, this "answer book" covers the gamut of real-life issues and problems faced by nurse managers in a variety of settings. The plethora of examples and lists and practical how-tos make this a unique contribution to the nursing management literature. In my years of working with nurse managers, I have found that this group wants information that makes sense and can be applied immediately and successfully. No one can guarantee success, of course, but this book absolutely delivers sensible, applicable information. Furthermore, because of the way it is organized, this book will be opened again and again. I wouldn't be surprised to see its pages become dogeared and thin from use.

The deep concern for the advancement of nurses demonstrated by these authors and many other nurse educators, researchers, and executives will make the difference in how the future of nursing unfolds. Knowledge and skill are power. The energy generated through education and skill building will fuel the development of nurse managers, the vanguard and pacesetters of 21st century health care delivery.

SUSAN C. ROE, DPA, RN

University of Phoenix
Phoenix, Arizona

Acknowledgments

WITH SPECIAL THANKS to the nursing managers and leaders at Harborview Medical Center, Seattle, Washington, and The University of Washington Medical Center, Seattle, Washington, for their participation in our surveys.

With gratitude to Michael Buelow, editor of the Arizona Nurse Times, for having a vision and encouraging us to be a part of that vision. Some of the answers included in this book originally appeared in column form as part of Michael's newspaper and have been refined, as we have, by the hand of experience. And to the respondents to the Arizona Nurse Times survey, who read our format and gave us suggestions and input. We appreciate your feedback and have incorporated it.

To all nurse managers and leaders everywhere—You're wonderful! Keep the faith *and* your sense of humor!

Introduction

IT'S DIFFICULT FOR us to remember the experiences of those first days as managers, but the feelings remain—exhilaration, fear, confusion, pride, anxiety. As the days lengthened into months, years, even decades, we began to understand (and even master) the complex role of nurse manager. How often, when we found a practical answer to a troubling situation, we vowed we'd find a method of sharing our experience with others. This book is our response to those promises to champion and sustain the brave along the way.

Perhaps you picked up this book looking for a "quick fix" to help you untangle the sticky web of people and systems hindering your management progress, something to clarify the muddle of management. We don't claim to possess the final answers to the specific questions for your individual struggle (nor the Holy Grail), but we have distilled complex concerns into logical, brief answers and suggestions based on our hard-earned experience. It is up to you to implement them! (Always there's a catch!)

As we have travelled, presented seminars, and consulted throughout the United States, we've been surprised by how many health care managers expressed the same concerns and needs as we've identified in our own careers as managers. Informal research in the form of questionnaires and focus groups has further identified priority topics. Based on our experience and research, we've answered many questions. We suggest you keep the answers handy to scan the steps for assistance when you're faced with "unanticipated adventures in management." If we've missed some, let us know and we'll include them in the next edition.

Some nurse managers may argue that we are attempting to oversimplify complicated, perplexing problems. We may be guilty as accused. However, we know that all of you were hired into your management roles because of your capabilities. We trust that you will use your personal competence to apply the volumes of material available to you in books on management theory, academic journals, and university classes to each situation you face. The theoretical background is essential, but often a few simple, step by step guidelines, distilling the art of leadership, are all that are necessary to provide additional confidence and direction.

We are here as your mentors, to guide and direct you. We have written these answers to you with humor and practicality, as we would to our favorite friends. The reasons? These answers represent a roadmap we wish we'd had. We believe that all of us in health care must begin to lead our teams to excellence. Who else will help ensure the quality of care for our parents, our children, for future generations?

The future of health care rests with each of us as leaders and managers. We have believed in ourselves, and we have found some tools to make management work. We are sharing them with you, supporting you in your mission.

I can tell you right now, there are no secrets. There's no mystery. There's only common sense.

OREN LYONS, FAITHKEEPER OF THE ONANDAGA NATION

CHAPTER 1

Now I'm a Hero?

WHETHER YOU ARE a seasoned professional or have recently added supervisory responsibilities to your role, you may be experiencing some conflicting emotions. Confusion about your role is often mixed with feelings of stress, uncertainty about your own abilities, as well as some excitement regarding the future and what you and your department will be able to accomplish.

In this section, we'll look at the transition from expert clinician in nursing to nursing management. The management tool chest will be opened and we'll examine the tools available for your use. We'll discuss the pervasive nature of change and chaos and how these will affect you and your work. Finally, you'll be reminded of your hero potential as a leader in your organization.

Hang in there! We think these answers will help you sort out your conflicts and help you feel better about being a manager.

We all live in suspense, from day to day, from hour to hour, in other words, we are the hero of our own story.

MARY MCCARTHY

Q #1 I've just become a nurse manager. Any suggestions that will make the change easier?

A Congratulations! This is an exciting, challenging, rewarding, and exhausting (we believe in reality) time in your career! But making the transition from clinician to manager is not an easy one, and will depend in part on a variety of factors. We are reminded of the story of the nurse who was asked by her manager if her future goals included a management position. The new nurse looked at her boss in shock and said, "Oh no! I want to stay in nursing!" You may at times feel as if you have left your profession for something quite different and that you are no longer a nurse. We hope that the following suggestions (indeed the whole book) will assist you and make the transition an easier one as you grow in your new position.

- Be clear about the expectations of the role that you now have. Asking what the staff expect of you is a good place to start. Brief one-to-one encounters with each member of the staff or a meeting, in which you ask staff members to describe what they need from you and how they expect you to function, will help to lay the foundation for your new position. You will also want to share your expectations of how you see yourself as their manager. This strategy can help to forestall those hasty judgments of unmet expectations that staff may be tempted to lay on you if you don't pass their acid test of management in the first ninety days. (Why doesn't she help do bed baths—she doesn't seem busy!) It will also let them know that you expect involvement from the staff (participative management) and is a dynamic way of sending the message that you value what they say!

- Review your image of yourself. Do you see yourself as the clinical expert? And do others see you in the clinical role as well? You may find that the staff expects you to be the best clinical support while being the leader as well. We suggest that this will be difficult to do, if you are to be a successful manager! (There are only so many hours in the day!) Your new role will require you to develop many talents and skills that were a part of your clinical expertise, but to apply them in a new way so that the people that work with you can be guided and supported to provide *their* best clinical skills to their patients. Are you ready to see yourself as a leader who happens to be a nurse, or are you looking to be a nurse who happens to be a leader? It is important to understand your own motives and expectations so that you don't take the path that leads only to frustration.

- First impressions are important. During the first weeks of your new job, everyone will be looking at you with a very critical eye. What you wear, where you are and when, what you say to anyone, will be observed and judged as you begin to develop your image and establish relationships. This spotlight may be friendly at first (some refer to it as the honeymoon period) and you will be able to make your best impression. Proceed with the idea that everyone wants you to succeed and not to fail, and concentrate on the little things.

- Pay attention to details, ask for input, say thanks, and remember people's names (especially your new boss)! As Harvey MacKay (1988, p. 155) says, "Little things don't mean a lot—they mean everything." People will remember (for a long time) the actions that you take during your first days. Use your new visibility wisely by being consistently aware of the important aspects of the personal touch. (We have an advantage here as nurses: we are generally more in tune to the caring side of life than our business counterparts.)

- Find a mentor. Just as when you were a new graduate nurse struggling to feel confident and to fit in, you need to connect with someone who is experienced in the management role and who demonstrates qualities that you would like to develop yourself. Meet with this person! Share your thoughts and find out if he or she is open to being available as a resource and an inspiration! (Who could turn this down?) See Question 10 for additional assistance.

- Focus on developing relationships that are built on respect, not on friendliness. We have seen many new managers knock themselves out doing things for their staff because they "want to be liked." Be wary of quickly running to solve a problem that a staff member brings to your door, hoping that person will "like" you more. Be wary too of your tendency to hold back in making requests of your staff "because they may not like me" or "will like me more if I do it myself and don't overburden them." Building trusting relationships does not mean becoming a friend, but being respected. This is a difficult issue to master because we all want to feel liked. If your relationship is based on being a friend to all of the staff members, how difficult will it be to resolve the conflict when their priorities do not agree with yours? The critical difference is respect. Once respect is developed, we suspect that people will like you as well.

- Be yourself. As time goes on, you will hear a great deal about management style and developing your own image. It's important that you do not let the title and position go to your head as you try to adopt a new persona to fit the role and you seek to become what you think others want you to be. Some people stop telling jokes, even though they have been known for their sense of humor in a tough situation. It's as if they now think the new position requires a more serious approach and they are never seen to crack a smile, much less laugh. This is a minor change compared to the more often seen tendency to become obsessed with the power and authority of the position, becoming the leader that rules with an iron fist. We repeat: Be yourself. It's your best asset and no doubt is the reason you were promoted in the first place.

> *Don't be afraid to take a big step if one is indicated. You can't cross a chasm in two small jumps.*
>
> DAVID LLOYD GEORGE

Q #2 I'm a clinical expert and I know how to use my clinical skills. Are the tools for management any different?

A Don't you wish they'd give you a working tool box for management, complete with instructions or a simple demonstration? You've felt comfortable with other tools in the clinical area—syringes, stethoscope, monitors, etc.—and are proud of the skills you have developed to use them. Now, will these tools do you any good?

This is such a wonderful story, that we're going to depart from our usual format a little bit to include it as it was told by one of our most inspirational leaders . . .

A long time ago there lived an elephant who decided to leave his herd in search of better tools to bring back, so that the herd, in seeing in his wisdom would then make him the leader. Starting out, he came upon a farmer using a large stick to break the ground. The elephant thought how much more efficient that would make him and so he asked the farmer to give him the stick. The farmer declined, saying he needed the stick for his work, but if the elephant would care to trade him his ears for the stick, he would do so. The elephant thought this over, and finding it a fair trade, he exchanged the ears for the stick.

Continuing on his journey, the elephant arrived at a fishing boat to watch the fishermen skillfully using a net. Thinking this to be a very handy tool to have, the elephant asked the fishermen for the net. The main fisherman was wise, and seeing a trade in the making, he offered the elephant the net in exchange for his tusks. Not needing the tusks, because he now had a stick, the elephant agreed to the trade.

Coming upon an old woman finishing a beautiful wool blanket, the elephant thought this would keep him warm at

*night. The woman was a tough trader and realizing how
much the elephant wanted the blanket, she agreed to exchange it for one of the elephant's feet, from which she
would make a table. The elephant agreed (after all, he had
four feet) and the trade was made.*

*Returning to his herd, the elephant eagerly shared his
new tools. The leader was dismayed, calling the traveler a
foolish elephant. "Your tusks would have lasted much
longer than that stick will. You will need help to use the net,
and while the blanket will keep you warm at night, you have
no ears to fan yourself in the hot summer days ahead. And
now, with only three feet, you cannot keep up with the
herd." And so, the elephant was left to live out his days
alone, no more like a man or a leader, but less of an elephant
in his search for the tools of the trade. (Personal communication, Dan Frank, CEO, Community Hospital, Phoenix,
Arizona, 1990)*

- Remember the elephant! You are in a different position now,
  not necessarily the one you were originally trained to do.
  The majority of us do not start out as managers but instead
  spend some time in staff positions performing our first career step. As a staff nurse, you were not trained to manage
  the medical/surgical department of a large hospital; you
  were not given the tools in your education to balance a budget, counsel and fire employees, or design a new waiting
  room for the patients who visit your department. You may
  be overwhelmed with frustration, feeling ill-equipped to do
  the job, and seeking new tools to assist you. Before you make
  any trades, remember the elephant in our story and read on.

- Why are you in this position? Unlike our elephant, if you are
  reading this book, you are no doubt already in a management position. What got you the promotion? When you feel
  frustration at its highest, remember that you were promoted
  for some very good reasons. The skills that you demon-

strated in performing your staff role—planning, organizing, leading, and controlling (yes, you do all that as a staff nurse)—are skills that will continue to serve you well in this new role of management. You do not need to trade these skills, which are a part of you, to become someone else, to become one of "them."

• Build on the same foundation. If the elephant had only realized that he could have become the leader by improving the skills he already had, he wouldn't be in the mess he created. By expanding your initial abilities, and not trying to trade them to become someone else, you can enhance your own tools of the trade and remain human in the process.

> *I would not give a fig for the simplicity this side of complexity, but I would give my life for the simplicity on the other side of complexity.*
>
> JUSTICE OLIVER WENDELL HOLMES

Q #3 How do I handle all this change?

A *Change is a fact of life in health care.* It is impossible to hold on to the status quo. Who would want to? Most of us would agree that there's a lot of room for improvement in our current system. Change is necessary to create a future that could include such dreams as fair and equal access to basic health care, comprehensive preventive care, streamlined treatment modalities, and keeping health care providers financially solvent. And when considering chaos, we'd like any organization that never experiences some chaos to write us as soon as possible. We'd love to make an onsite visit!

In our solution, we'll discuss two basic concepts essential for coping with change and chaos. First is the necessity of exploring the qualities of change and chaos in more detail and examining our attitudes toward them. Second is the need to determine your "constants"—the rocks you'll cling to when the winds of change and chaos whip through your department or organization.

- Recognize it's futile to run from change. Learn to embrace it. If you try to dig in your heels, you'll just leave your boots in the muck when you are forced to go with the flow.

- Review several change theories. Determine where you are, where your staff members fit into the models, and how they react to change. There are many good theories about how to best reduce resistance to change, and these *always* recommend inclusion of all the participants in the change in the early stages. We recommend Jennifer James's discussion of change as a window. It's positive and practical. She outlines six steps:

  1. Death rattle (you deny need to change)

  2. The window opens (you see an opportunity)

  3. Exploration (you explore the options)

  4. Tumble through (you willingly take the plunge, or you are forced to make the change)

  5. Landing on your feet (you begin to adjust)

  6. Sharing (you tell everyone about the benefits)

  As James states, "The magic is in the attention you are willing to give the windows; the pain is in the avoidance."

- Reassess your expectations about chaos. (Chaos equals unanticipated, stressful events.) Although all of us hope to lead departments that run like clockwork, never experiencing a glitch in the machinery, think about it. Is it reasonable to expect no glitches when you are working with 100 plus people from many different disciplines and with patients and families that are experiencing the most traumatic or stressful events in their lives? We are talking about a miracle where there isn't a bit of chaos from time to time. (For those of us striving for "zero defects" in our quality management program, this does not mean quit striving. Just don't become immobilized if chaos rears its ugly head now and then.)

- Given that the people part of the business will always create some challenges, do all that you can to make the environment as positive as possible for your work group. Identify and remove the barriers that exist to getting the job done as smoothly as possible. When the winds and waves of change try to throw you, the ever-constant rock must be the *mission* and *vision* of your department, and the knowledge that you are there to support and facilitate your staff's accomplishment of that mission.

- Keep your own constants forever in front of you by writing them, talking about them, visualizing them. Right now, quickly assess whether you can articulate the following:

  ☐ your own motivation for being in this role

  ☐ a clear mission and vision for your department

  ☐ a set of behaviorally defined performance standards

  ☐ a plan or program for fixing the problems, removing the barriers, and keeping people constantly communicating

- Since we must expect change and occasional chaos, recognize that your own stress level will depend on your inner expectations. If you begin to believe that you are adaptable to change and that some chaos keeps you and your group on your toes, ever watchful for new opportunities for growth, your working environment will be a much more positive place. Your staff will slowly begin to share your attitude. You will experience eustress (or good stress) instead of the artery clogging, blood pressure elevating bad stress. Besides, spending time continually complaining about all the bad problems in health care or in your department (woe is us!) will create a detour of time and energies that could be devoted to adaptation, creation of better alternatives, and the shaping of a better future!

> *Avoiding danger is no safer in the long run than outright exposure. The fearful are caught as often as the bold.*
>
> HELEN KELLER

Q #4
I'm just trying to keep my head above water, and you've said I have to be a hero. How can I be Supernurse and Supermanager as well?

A Have you looked over your shoulder yet to see if anyone has discovered you're really the same person you were before you took on this job and this title? Whether it's your first day on the job, or you've been "in charge" for a long time, there are times you wish you'd never accepted the position. At some point, it becomes clear that you are accountable for everything in your department, from the function of the visitors' toilet to the quality of the care or service you provide.

Believe it or not, the day you changed your name badge, you became a potential hero. The hero myth is a part of our human growth and development, symbolizing the individual's struggle from youth to mature adulthood. In our society, leaders and managers are cultural heroes who have been somehow magically endowed with courage, strength, self-sacrifice, and humility. People will look to you for these qualities. Pretty daunting and actually downright scary, right? So how can you discover your own hero potential and remain in management?

1. Determine your own motivation for accepting a management job. Is it for prestige? The farther up the ladder a person goes, the larger possible view of the person's derrière. The thrill of a new office, or even more money, pales when there isn't a purpose to what you do. Or, is it because you knew you could do a better job than some of your previous bosses? Don't be too humble with yourself, because this is a great reason for being a manager. You will be able to be a better boss if you remain in touch with your own failings and continue to learn and grow. Is it because you feel called to lead, to inspire others to help create a better health care system? If so, we need you!

2. Having determined your own purpose for being in management, hold onto those intentions every day. It is essential to your sanity to be in touch with your personal reasons for accepting this potentially exciting and fulfilling position when stressors and challenges proliferate.

3. The way you perform as a manager is fundamental to the successful functioning of your group. It is within your power to make or break the product or service you are creating, to empower or imprison your staff, and to lead the organization to excellence or failure. You *will* make a difference, either way you choose to play it.

4. Management is a challenging, creative, and highly rewarding profession in itself. Recognize that your worth as a person is not hinging on whether or not you continue to perform the technical functions of your profession on a daily basis. Your job is to support, facilitate, remove roadblocks, communicate, give feedback, mentor, dream, and inspire. Your department will appreciate it

when you realize management is extremely valuable to the organization. (Our staff members were very happy when we came to terms with the significance of management work!)

5. Remember those mythical qualities of courage, strength, self-sacrifice, and humility? Develop these qualities and you will be a superleader! It takes self-awareness, asking for feedback, and the openness for change and growth. (You won't even need a telephone booth for changing into your outfit, because it will be a part of who you are.)

The final test of a leader is that he leaves behind him in other men the conviction and the will to carry on.

WALTER LIPPMAN

REFERENCES

James, J. (in press). *Thinking in the future tense.* New York: Simon & Schuster.

MacKay, H. (1988). *Swim with the sharks without being eaten alive.* New York: Random House, Inc.

CHAPTER 2

Am I a Manager or a Leader or Both?

WE'VE ATTEMPTED TO gently answer the first questions asked by people recently taking on supervisory roles. (We thought that being gentle and kind would be a welcome experience for most new managers!) Before we get to the nitty gritty questions, we'd like to build on a few more of the basic ideas of management. What's the difference between management and leadership, and who will know which function you're attempting to execute? How important are the values you hold dear in the total scheme of things? Is it possible for managers to adapt their style to different situations, and how does one keep in touch with what's really happening at the point of service to the client? Many of us also worry about the impact of our image as we manage/lead. We'll discuss all these issues in this chapter.

Dwight Eisenhower used to discuss his leadership style by using a piece of household twine. He'd display the string and say: "Pull it, and it will follow anywhere you wish. Push it, and it will go nowhere at all."

Q #5   Am I a leader or a manager? What's the difference?

A It's become popular for management texts to speak to this issue, noting there is an important difference that must be identified so that individuals are clear about the path they are following. For clarification, we go to the experts themselves. In their popular book, *Leaders: The Strategies for Tak-*

ing Charge, Warren Bennis and Burt Nanus (1985, p.21) define managers as those who "do things right" and leaders as those who "do the right thing." This sounds like a catchy little phrase to confuse the issue, and yet it is a very simplistic way of explaining the differences of the two roles. Too often we have found that little attention is paid to the differences and the assumption is made that the manager is, of course, the leader.

A good manager of any hospital unit or department (we hope you've had the opportunity to work with one) will have the correct staffing ratios, budget reports completed monthly with variances explained, and will organize the work flow by delegating tasks to the appropriate personnel. The result of "doing things right" (good management) will be a smoothly run unit with relative stability. Not a bad achievement (and no small task) in today's health care environment.

On the other hand, a good leader will focus on identifying new directions and new approaches to old problems or old solutions in order to change the environment for the better. This often involves risk taking and the ability to sell a vision that will be supported by the staff. Traditionally, the chief executive and presidential positions are synonymous with leadership. We're not asking you to assume presidential authority, but to take steps to identify the differences in the two roles. It's not simply a question of style, as much as it is a clarification of one focus versus the other. Have you ever worked for someone who was quite content to keep things the way they were and spent all energy of the staff directed at achieving a well-run unit that maintained status quo? How did you and the rest of the staff feel? Frustrated at the sameness, or safe in the sense that nothing ever changes around here?

In your position now, there may be times when you change from one focus to another, because your position challenges you to provide a vision for the future as well as to keep the department on course. Your personal combination of skills, values, motivation, and experience will determine which role you are generally most comfortable with, and which hat you wear the most often. Our sense is that your staff needs both, and today's manager exhibits leadership as well as management skills.

1. Identify your personal approach to problems. Are you a problem solver or one who likes to challenge the system and look at a situation from a new angle? Do you feel more comfortable with predictable outcomes, or do you like the excitement of unpredictability? Perhaps there's a "rebel" among your group who always proposes a novel approach to daily operational problems, and the staff support his or her ideas, even though you're the boss. How do you react to that individual? (Would you like to silence him or her for good, or do you thank God he or she's there to make your job more interesting?)

2. Define your relations with others. Generally speaking, managers prefer to work with other people (after all, management is defined as getting work done through others). Leaders, however, often find themselves in the position of trailblazing and prefer to go it alone. When you have a new idea, or an old one that you're recycling, do you look to others for involvement and support, or do you make the pitch yourself?

3. Assess your ability to perform the following skills:

   ☐ Challenging the process: similar to your personal approach to problem solving, being adept at this skill means you are comfortable with being a "maverick" and choosing a new path or supporting a new method proposed by someone else on your staff.

   ☐ Inspiring a shared vision: whether it's your new vision

(leader) or the company's mission, is everyone in your boat rowing in the same direction (manager)? Management requires that many people operate efficiently in different positions with varied responsibilities. Directing this process and achieving harmony among the troops is essential for successful management.

☐ Encouraging the heart: do you celebrate success? (We'll ask this often—it's important!) What importance do you attach to recognition of good work? (See Question 25.) Being manager requires a certain amount of cheerleading to maintain a coordinated effort.

☐ Enabling others to act: are you comfortable delegating opportunities to staff members for a team approach to getting the job done, or do you resist delegation, preferring to achieve your own standard?

4. Strive for a blend of managerial and leadership qualities in yourself. The leader pilots the course, setting new directions for the crew to follow, complemented by the manager, the very necessary navigator who keeps the craft running with a watchful eye on the fuel and today's weather conditions. The result is an excellent partnership, whether combined in one individual working as today's new leader/manager, or shared by members of the team who are committed to reaching new horizons.

Good management without leadership . . . an organization that looks good while going nowhere.

AUTHOR UNKNOWN

Q #6   What's in a mission statement anyway?

A   As a manager, we're certain (reasonably) that you have read the mission statement of your organization. Hopefully, you've not only read it, but had an opportunity to participate in the development or revision of the current statement. Why do we say that? We all know the generic format of everyone's mission in health care goes something like this: "To provide the highest quality patient care in the most cost effective manner possible." Given that we all share this common goal, what's the importance of a mission statement to any organization and, ultimately, to you and the members of your unit? Depending on your facility, the mission statement is either the cornerstone upon which performance is based, or merely a narrative serving as the face sheet for the policy book. The determining factor can be found in the lines that follow the common goal; those *guiding principles* or *values* that should outline the facility's priorities for defining and achieving quality care.

There is a growing trend in management today (as organizations gradually shift from a bureaucratic value system to a more humanistic/democratic system) that places value on the complex needs of all individuals in their relationship to work, the organization, and their environment. Values, those general, enduring beliefs about what's truly important in life, shape our behavior and are beginning to be identified by progressive leadership (that's YOU!) as the foundation for successful management.

What does all this mean for you as a manager of health care today? How can you make the mission of your organization real for your staff, and important to your management success? Here are some answers:

- Understand your organization's mission. This sounds pretty simple, but have you taken the time to READ the statement that adorns your hallway (usually by the elevator) or forms the front page to those weighty tomes, the Policy and Procedures manuals? Having a clear understanding of this document is the important first step in determining if, as an employee, YOUR values will be supported.

- What are your values? Yes, this means that you must also take some time to identify your own personal philosophy. We have found that many people tend to overlook this step, thinking it's too obvious or esoteric, and not necessary to doing the job. By now, you know we couldn't disagree more, as many of the answers in this book bring you back to your set of values, your sense of goals, to clarify the meaning in your working life. Failing to take the time to complete this personal introspection means that many people operate on instinct, making decisions based on their feeling at that moment. This can lead to confusion, inconsistency, interpersonal conflict, and conflict with the organization as a whole. Who can follow that kind of management?

- Check for alignment of your values with those of the organization. For instance, in the pursuit of quality care, what does your agency emphasize? Education may be stated as the focus, physician support and collaboration may have been identified, and employee development/recognition through participation listed as a primary value. Or the focus may be solely on business development, making little or no mention of the employee's role in achieving this growth. Is this congruent with your personal values? As Dr. Sid Simon, ethicist and author, advises in the Diann Uustal book (1985, p.138), "Do what you value. Value what you do." Finding an organization that truly is in agreement with and supports your personal values is essential to your management success. If you don't have that agreement, the feeling will be worse than wearing a pair of ill-fitting shoes. The blisters that you get will only serve to make you more disagreeable and discontent, and your staff will respond accordingly!

- Make the mission real for your staff. Our guess is that a considerable amount of effort went into the drafting of this document. Is it available for the employees? Is it something that is talked about and truly used as the benchmark for everything that is done in the organization? We have found that it is not unusual for employees to know about the existence of such a document, but to also question its value and to have some degree of skepticism about the reality of it. Spending time discussing this at a staff meeting, making the mission statement part of your lounge bulletin board, and having a committee develop supporting statements that are specific to your unit are good strategies for making the mission more visible. Utilizing the mission as the framework for making decisions and solving employee conflicts will also make this more than just a pretty piece of paper that marketing dreamed up.

- Learn the process for the revision/updating of the mission statement. Is this a process that can be accessed by employees? (We hope so!) Who has the final approval of any changes? Employee involvement will help to create the sense of importance intended by this document, which is the very framework of your organization. (And you thought it was just something to read while waiting for the elevator!)

> *Nursing's values—commitment, responsibility, service— are about to become the hallmarks of the successful person and business of the next century. Forty years ago, Albert Einstein said "Let us strive not to be people of success, but people of value." Today we seem finally to be learning that people of value are people of success. Nurses have the history, the tradition, and the values . . .*
>
> LEAH CURTIN

Q #7   Should I adapt my leadership style according to the situation?

A You've been the manager of the cardiovascular department in your hospital for the last six months. Busy in your office interviewing a secretarial candidate, you hear a loud voice outside the door bellowing, "My wife's room has been filthy throughout her hospitalization and the air conditioner is on HIGH all the time. There is constant noise from all the machines! Can't you make the environment better for her? She's not getting well because of this!" You are aware of which staff members are working in the outer office and that they may be able to deal with this situation.

Do you decide to (a) continue with the interview and allow the staff in the office to help this person? They've recently discussed handling of complaints and are very sensitive to the stress experienced by the patients' families. You are confident they will hold true to your department's values of customer satisfaction and the dignity of the individual; or (b) excuse yourself from the secretarial candidate, open the door, and intervene yourself? You are aware that handling complaints sensitively is a weak area in your staff members' development, and that they'll need some coaching in this process by watching you work with this irate person.

If you answered both a and b, congratulations! You are aware of the fact that your leadership choices depend on the situation; most significantly, on the characteristics of your team and their development. Consider great political or religious leaders. Their personal characteristics are varied: from the more quiet, low-key manager trusted for his or her infallible judgment to the flamboyant orator inspiring the flock to action with his zeal. No matter where your personality falls within the spectrum, you can be successful if you are willing to flex your responses in a manner that matches the needs of the group you lead.

- Develop an understanding of your most common leadership style. Use one of the self-assessment tests available in management literature, but supplement it with a frank feedback discussion with some trusted staff, peers, and your supervisor.

- Broaden your ability to adapt by developing additional leadership styles. (It would be great if all managers took method acting lessons to develop the ability to change behavior instantly based on a given situation.) Charades within the management group can be great fun and can be a learning experience for all. For example: Managers could act out real responses to especially difficult situations in their departments, and then how they *wish* they would have managed these situations. A great byproduct will be the managers' ability to see each other as human and to ask each other for help in the future.

- Get to know the strengths and weaknesses of each staff member as well as the group as a team. (See our answers on performance evaluation and coaching, Questions 25 and 27 for concrete suggestions.) Each shift may have different characteristics based on their experience level and training. Assessment of the group is done by listening, observing, and by looking at quality data. Do many ask for more specific direction, or are they offended if you seem too controlling? Do they welcome tasks you have delegated, energetically tackling the project with very little need for guidance?

- Match the characteristics of the staff with the situation and your behavior. Are they new, inexperienced, and unsure? They'll need detailed direction during a time of stress and change. Are they feeling more comfortable with their roles and job descriptions? They will need coaching, gentle guidance with open, two-way communication. When staff are more knowledgeable and motivated, you may be needed to provide recognition, facilitate problem solving, and give feedback, always helping articulate the vision or broad goals.

- Major problems have occurred due to mismatching of management behavior with the group's needs. But early recognition of the misdiagnosis of the readiness of the group to take on a task or project allows for continual adjustment of the plan. Just as leader/managers expect their staff to recognize problems and redirect their course, the staff will expect the leaders to supervise the navigation.

- Be gentle with yourself. Being a savvy manager takes some time. Usually the most savvy managers have risked a lot, made many mistakes, and learned from them. They become more and more experienced at matching their behavior with the needs of the group in the given situation.

> *Let whoever is in charge keep this simple question in her head (NOT, how can I always do this right thing myself, but) how can I provide for this right thing always to be done?*
>
> FLORENCE NIGHTINGALE

Q #8   I can't seem to get out of my office! Can I effectively manage if I don't get out and around?

A   "Well, what would *she* know about it? She hasn't left her office for days!" It seems impossible to keep in touch with what's happening within your unit or organization when the paperwork is falling off your desk, the phone is ringing off the hook, and your calendar is bulging with meetings!

Think about how you assess your patients, how visually encountering them and talking with them yields immeasurable amounts of sensory data that can't be obtained by reading a chart. We often speak of *knowing* our patients or peers. Being around and being involved with them is our route to *knowing*. Talking face-to-face with your teenager for just a few minutes will reveal a problem at school, a homework, social, financial, or transportation issue, needing parental intervention. (Remember when YOUR parents asked you to come into their bedroom to say goodnight when you got home from a date? They had several objectives besides a good night's sleep.) Although parental intervention may sometimes seem geared to potential punishment, it may parallel managerial involvement through the objectives of *avoiding developing problems, providing real-time guidance,* and *recognizing challenges and trends* that beg for immediate or future attention.

- Despite the seemingly insurmountable mountain of information, keep as technically current as you possibly can. If you are a unit or department manager, subscribe to the pertinent journals and take time to read them. (OK, if you haven't yet been able to allocate the time to read, at least scan the pertinent articles!) The respect of the clients, physicians, other departments, and your staff depends on your ability to be involved intelligently in clinical decisions. (There are now journal scanning services available in most areas.) Your ability to plan proactively for the future as a leader depends on your understanding of trends and political and social issues as well.

- Whatever your administrative level, *make rounds* in your facility. Talk with patients, physicians, staff. They will appreciate your interest. (After all, they've been secretly wondering how you can know anything about operations without being there from time to time.)

- As you make rounds or just chat, you'll find that you can identify trends and potential problems much more quickly from your vantage point than by all the filtered information you'll receive from your advisors or specified team members. Your designated "stool pigeons" may think they know what you want to hear, and will provide just that.

- Find a way to have contact with all the shifts, if your organization runs 24 hours per day. Even though your calendar is totally booked, it is possible to plan each month to do some of your work during evening or night hours. There's a different atmosphere during different shifts, and experiencing it is fun! (Yes, we even mentioned *fun!* If you aren't having fun yet, consult a career advisor, head hunter, or Question 72.)

- You'll discover that *they* (the workers in your organization) are wonderful people with varied personalities and strengths. *They* are much easier to work with during negotiations or other conflicts when you *know them* and what they do.

- Observe. Use all your senses as a client or patient may. Put yourself in the role of a surveyor. Ask questions. Look for the good, the fine, the outstanding, embryonic legends. Use your data for improving systems and for discovering and broadcasting stars and successes.

> *The growing American characteristically defends himself against anxiety by learning not to become too involved.*
>
> EDGAR Z. FRIEDENBERG

Q #9   I hear all this stuff about dressing for success, having the right accessories, being seen with the right people. Is all this really important?

A Afraid so. We live in a highly visual society, where judgments are made instantly on the basis of how someone LOOKS. We're not saying that it's fair, but we are saying that because of our current cultural emphasis, attention to style is extremely important. Having said that, we bet you could use some pointers about what we mean regarding creating your own image.

- Take a look in the mirror. Does what you see inspire confidence? Does the image project a capable, caring, and competent individual that we would feel comfortable following? We're not just talking about good grooming here, although that goes without saying. We *are* looking for an upright posture, a smile on your face, and an expression that says you expect to be treated with respect. Droopy shoulders, coupled with a frown or a stern look, speak loudly about your self perception. Before you don that business suit with the matching classic jewelry and black (brown or burgundy is acceptable too) briefcase, make sure that your posture and body language are in tune to the message that you want to convey. This simple strategy, stand up straight and face the world with a smile (on your face and a song in your heart, remember the words to that old song? or are we dating ourselves?) will be much more effective than spending hundreds of dollars on a new suit. (However, if you need an excuse to buy a new suit, we'll be happy to provide one!)

- Take a look at your closet. We know we just said that your physical stance was more important, but the clothes will also make a statement about your image. Dress codes may require you to wear specific articles of clothing; men may be required to wear ties at all times; women may or may not be allowed to wear slacks. It is hard to believe that, as we approach the twenty first century, we still have clothing restrictions, but that only reminds us how important the issue is. If you have relative freedom at your facility, we recommend the conservative, business approach to dressing. Make sure it fits, that it matches, and that it's clean for starters. Stick to classic, simple lines, saving the ruffles and loud ties for somewhere else. If you're not sure about all this, go shopping with someone who is, someone who always looks well put together and whom you would like to look like. You don't need to spend a fortune on the latest designs, but the uniform you wore as a staff nurse is certainly no longer your main attire. A lab coat is always appropriate for clinical areas, but best left behind for the administrative meeting of the month.

- Take a look at your office. We suspect that you don't spend a lot of time there (you're busy out on the unit getting to know your folks and managing by walking around) but the times that you and someone else are in the office make this an important part of your image as well. This is an opportunity to make a statement about yourself, in the most positive manner possible. We worry about the office where the desk top can't be seen, where the file drawers are stuffed and open and there are posters on the wall, or nothing at all. Sure, you're busy! But find some time on a Saturday to come in and straighten up the place, adding your special touch that says this is your office. Some people will put their degrees on the wall (framed please), a favorite painting, or a few framed photos of special events. Whatever you choose, make certain it's hung neatly and that it portrays the message you want people to receive when they walk into your office for the first time. We caution against cartoon posters and stuffed animals that you may have collected; people may wonder if you are mature enough to be there when the going gets really tough. We remember one nurse manager who never believed in the importance of appearance and consequently had an office that looked like a war zone. Staff would timidly approach her office, standing at the door because there was never a place to sit. They freely talked about her inability to get organized and to hold it together, often resisting her ideas and sharing the attitude that "nothing ever gets done around here." Cleaning up her office one Saturday afternoon (it was a New Year's resolution), she found a new attitude from her staff on Monday morning. So many people commented on the difference in her office that she was amazed. She'll never forget (we're sure) the one nurse who summed it all up by saying, "Now, maybe we'll see some action around here!"

- Be aware of emotional displays. Yes, the new management literature abounds with the idea that it's OK to be real at work, that it's even OK to cry. And, as nurses, we certainly know and understand the value of sharing feelings during those especially difficult moments. It's important that your staff sees you as real, but choose your moments wisely and privately so that you are also known to have self control and are not easily overwhelmed. We advise strongly against emotional displays around your boss! Calm demeanor in crises will instill confidence in your abilities.

- You lose points for smoking and being overweight. (Sorry, but that's the way it is.) One of the best ways a leader can lead is by example, so be sure that yours is one that you will want people to follow. It was no different when you were counseling the congestive heart failure (CHF) patient about the need to lose twenty pounds. The message is harder to believe if your uniform is bulging at the seams! The same is true for smoking. People do not want to see health care providers indulging in a practice that is so blatantly unhealthy. Control these habits so that your image does *not* state, "Do as I say, not as I do."

- Keep in shape. Take care of yourself (yes, we are saying this again, because we know how you are) so that you do not appear tired or worn out from the demands of your position. This *is* a demanding role and we are not asking you to portray super human qualities. However, a leader is much more inspiring who is full of energy, does not have bags under the eyes and a look of shell shock, and doesn't drag through the day. So take care that those long days are not taking an excessive toll and undermining all of your efforts because you look like something the cat dragged in. Even on airplanes we are advised to put the oxygen mask on ourselves *before* our children. Take care of yourself first so that you can lead the rest of us to achieve the vision you have for nursing!

Go put your creed into your deed.

RALPH WALDO EMERSON

REFERENCES

Bennis, W. & Nanus, B. (1985). *Leaders: The strategies for taking charge.* New York: Harper & Row.

Uustal, D.B. (1985). *Values and ethics in nursing: From theory to practice.* East Greenwich, RI: Educational Resources in Nursing and Holistic Health.

CHAPTER 3

▬▬▬▬▬▬

How Can I Create a Personal Network?

MANAGERIAL JOBS CAN be very lonely. No longer are you "one of the crowd." It's generally not good strategy to share all of your feelings or thoughts freely with your staff. So, how can you find the support and mentorship you need? Who is available to answer your questions and direct you, without giving the impression of naiveté or ignorance? How can professional organizations be of help? What about power and politics? Does our organizational culture and my gender play a part in the way I do my job? The issues we cover in this chapter may be some of the most delicate, as we tackle subjects you won't find in most management handbooks. Adapting our solutions to your situation will require some prior thought, and implementing the ideas will challenge your creativity and finesse. Go for it!

> *Relationships are like pressures that push you in 36 directions of the compass. But, as in a crowded streetcar, if you learn how to maintain your balance against the weights, you might arrive at yourself.*

> DIANA CHANG

Q #10 How can I find peer support or a mentor? (Or, "Nobody loves me, everybody hates me, guess I'll go eat worms!")

A You are definitely in the middle! Some of your staff members are angry, your clients or public are unhappy, the families are belligerent, your boss is asking the impossible, your family wants you to wear your name badge at home so they can remember your name! Where can you find relief and support? How can you find help for survival of this difficult time?

- No, you are not crazy for feeling stressed out. There is not a manager or leader in history that has never felt frustrated and alone. The very nature of the role predisposes you to these feelings: you are committed, accountable, caring. Your burning desire is to motivate and lead others to a better future. The team doesn't always follow in the prompt manner you hope to witness. Few organizations "organically" respond to change with timely adaptation. Not enough bosses are open and encouraging. Feeling down is a normal part of a challenging job. And, remember, if there were no problems and all staff members were self-motivated and coached themselves on to excellence, many more managers would be out of work!

- Before (or after or during) the tears, think about the peer relationships that you have been building since the first day of your job. (A note here to male managers: yes, it is OK to cry, preferably in private! There is a trend now toward the "feminine" leadership style, which includes "getting in touch with your feelings.") Have your noticed a friendly person with whom you feel comfortable? Look for someone who is able to keep a confidence and has some potential for having been in a similar situation. Often those in peer or lateral positions may have some wise words based on what has worked for them in similar circumstances or may be able to listen sympathetically. Touch bases with this person. Ask whether he or she has time for lending an ear and giving you some advice.

- Be certain not to reveal confidential information when you are discussing problems. Self-revelation when emotions run high may be seen as a negative in the future. Building trust with peers occurs in a gradual manner, as private disclosures are respectfully and mutually kept. You may wish to consult with someone in a parallel position in a former organization if they have been previously trustworthy.

- Find a mentor, whether within or outside of your organization, who is more experienced and has wisdom and maturity built from overcoming obstacles in his or her professional life. Discuss your perception of the work situation.

- Take time to be alone to think and plan. (See Question 39 about fighting fires.)

- Read as much as you can about management. (This book, for example, gives you the benefit of quick and concise information to get you started on the right path to a better work life.)

- Plan for some social times for peer support. Often, getting away to a workshop with some of your colleagues can be tremendously supportive.

- Re-examine your reasons for being in management, for choosing your profession. Recognize that your daily contribution is extremely valuable to many other people—staff, patients, the organization, physicians, and other health care workers.

- You aren't perfect; you are in a continual pattern of growth and renewal. You don't expect the impossible of your team, don't expect the impossible of yourself.

> *The firmest friendships have been formed in mutual adversity, as iron is most strongly united by the fiercest flame.*
>
> CHARLES CALEB COLTON

Q #11 How do I get along better with my boss?

A What does your boss think of you? What kind of mood is he or she in today and how will that affect his or her response to the bad news you have? Why is your boss always "on your case?" Does your supervisor ever give you feedback when it's not time for your yearly performance review?

Recent surveys across the country demonstrate that how an employee relates (or doesn't relate) to his or her manager is one of the top five stress producers in employment. No matter what the position, or how well we are implementing self-governing teams, we all answer to a higher level of manager, from staff positions on up the organizational chart. (Even the CEO answers to the Board!)

Like it or not, the relationship you establish with your manager can make the difference in your working environment, your attitude, and your career. If you accept the fact that this managerial relationship has a potential for stress or success, it seems reasonable that time spent developing the relationship would be well invested. Successful people do realize this, and do not assume that the burden of getting along, of establishing communication, belongs solely to the manager.

We're not advocating politicking or brown-nosing your boss in order to get on his or her "good side." Consider an honest, upfront focus to the needs, concerns, and goals of another human being. (Yes, this person is human and happens to be in a key position in terms of your employment!) Just as in all human relations, "You get your change back in the same currency you pay." Attention focused on understanding your manager's style and expectations will be well worth the effort.

• Analyze your perception of management. Is your perception one of us versus them? Or are you a front line manager caught in the squeeze play between staff and administration, looking at your boss as too far removed from the "real issue" to be supportive? Knowing where you're coming from helps you to be aware of possible prejudices and value judgments you may be making regarding your boss.

- Learn about your boss's world. We often assume we know the answers to this question—the boss always talks about the budget, company goals, changing compensations from payors, and endless meetings. But what are the personal objectives this manager has for your department (or unit) and what pressures is he or she under to achieve them? What is your boss's definition of fun, success, work? Have you asked?

- Get to know your boss's style. Just like you, your boss has a preferred method of communication. Does he or she like long, detailed reports in writing, or a verbal account on a daily basis? Ask for specific direction, explaining your desire to meet his or her needs. Does your supervisor want to know every detail of your workday, or are you given lots of space, to the point where you question if anyone from the top is interested at all? We all have different styles of management, generally based on personality traits and the demands of the role we play. Being aware of this style, and working with it (by having the information ready when needed) can cure those feelings of resentment and potential misunderstanding.

- Communicate your expectations and ask for clear and measurable performance standards for your own role. Keeping expectations to yourself is an ambiguous game that even the best manager can't win. Clarifying your needs and perceptions of your boss's role will eliminate such unhappy scenes as: *"You're* the supervisor—you're supposed to *know* when I need help!" (Remember this is your boss, not a parent, and we think you would hate to hear this from a member of your team!)

- Treat your manager as a person. Give positive feedback and express appreciation for his or her support. Relationship building (and maintenance) is a two way street in all cases, and no less so because the person involved happens to be your supervisor. Active participation on your part can go a long way in establishing a productive working arrangement that is mutually satisfying.

> *Always communicate unto the other guy that which you would want him to communicate unto you if the positions were reversed.*
>
> AARON GOLDMAN

Q #12 I'd like to avoid the Watergate syndrome. How can I maintain my self-respect and integrity and that of my staff?

A It's bound to happen. Despite all your good intentions, it's possible that there is a practice going on within your department that doesn't fit within your ethical framework nor dovetail with your mission. Your trusted staff may tell you that they *assumed* you knew, and that you were just looking the other way. It's difficult to think that you may have given them the message that some dishonesty may be OK. After all, we don't always tell the *whole* truth about everything, do we?

- When you encounter an ethical problem, calmly meet with your staff members and discuss your concerns. Discuss *why* their decision to change policy could be detrimental to (for example) patient coverage, communication with physicians, productivity, and the plan to improve staff ratios during peak activity times. Describe your disappointment clearly, without pointing fingers and raging with righteous indignation. If you do, no one will tell you about a problem again for fear of incurring your wrath.

- Be honest with your employees regarding your own feelings and values. Be certain by what you communicate to them, verbally and nonverbally, that ethical standards will be followed. This means that there is serious discussion, no winking of the eye or crossed fingers to show you don't *really* mean it! (We are convinced that if this happened more frequently in our government, there would be less "sleaze.")

- Admit it when you have made a mistake. "I am sorry that I gave you the impression that rudeness to other departments was OK. I meant to tell you that I understand why you *feel* like being rude back to them, but it's not OK to sink to that communication style." Be public about it. This allows your team members to know they aren't expected to be perfect either.

- Keep lines of communication open so that there are not secrets. Most of us become uncomfortable with secrets that are devious in nature. Using the principles learned in management by walking around (Tom Peters, 1987) (Question 8) will help you be more aware of potential problems.

- Accept that as manager/leader, *you are accountable* for the behavior of your team. You aren't able to avoid all the problems, but when they occur, you must do something to correct them and to avoid them in the future. You must also recognize that when your staff does something illegal, immoral, or unethical, there *may be* ways you have contributed to the impression that their behavior may be "OK if you don't get caught." Think about whether you could have avoided this behavior if you had picked up on clues more quickly, and then act on this in the future.

- As leader, continue to communicate the group vision and mission. The mission will certainly communicate noble values, and these should be supported with clear ethical standards. Be certain everyone has a copy of (and has read) your profession's ethical code (for example, the International or ANA code of ethics). Don't pass up an opportunity to point out the ethical standards you and your team advocate.

Don't compromise yourself. You are all you've got.

JANIS JOPLIN

Q #13 We seem to do things one way around here, and if I try to suggest something different, people question me. What's going on?

A What's going on is a display of "organizational culture." Sounds like a pricey lab test, but it's really the concept of what an organization is in terms of its philosophies, values, beliefs, and attitudes that are commonly shared by the employees. Consider the following examples:

Susan Carter had been a staff nurse at a small community hospital for six years. She left to join the staff of a much larger metropolitan hospital, hoping for new opportunities. Less than a year later, she returned to the smaller facility, claiming she "just didn't fit in" at such a big place.

Kim Rogers had been with the same corporate hospital for three years. Believing in stability, after he received his graduate degree he applied for several management positions within the corporation. His frustration grew as he was repeatedly passed over for positions he sought; they were instead filled by applicants from outside the hospital. Seems that promoting from within was not the way things were done at Corporate Hospital.

Whether you are conscious of it or not (we recommend that you are), the place where you work has a "culture" of its own. Understanding that culture can be a positive part of your personal network. It can also be a major component in determining why your performance is successful and feels right or, when you're not successful, why it feels like you're swimming upstream.

- Take a closer look around the place where you work. How do people dress? Can you ignore the dress code, or is it strictly enforced? Is there a slogan to describe the organization's mission? Are titles used? Are there status symbols that are easily identified? (Do all the managers carry a clipboard or a planning calendar with them everywhere?)

- Describe the atmosphere where you work, both on your unit and in the facility in general. What does it *feel* like overall to be there? Would you describe the atmosphere as family oriented, high-tech and impersonal, corporate or business directed, driven by competition, or filled with team spirit?

- Listen to the phrases used, particularly in the orientation of new employees. Are slogans used, such as "Working Together the Memorial Way"? How often do you hear, "We always do it this way," when explaining to a new employee the current procedures on your unit?

- Analyze how change occurs in your organization. Is a new idea supported, encouraged, even expected? Or is there a wall of resistance to any new ideas, because the "Memorial Way" has always worked? We often overlook the clues around us that make up and describe the culture of the organization we've chosen to work in. When things get difficult, we're not sure why and may not consider the very idea of cultural compatibility. In our examples above, employees made decisions without considering the impact of each unique environment and whether it would fit with their goals. Knowing the practice at Corporate Hospital is to value outside resources in order to bring new life to management should cause Kim Rogers serious consideration when planning to stay there several years. Likewise, a major move from a small, "family" environment to a larger, possibly impersonal setting should be carefully considered before the transfer is made (by Susan or you).

- Consider your new employees. Are they suffering from "culture shock"? During your interviews, you probably look for someone who is not only skilled, but someone who will fit in with the rest of the group. It's natural to want to belong, to feel connected, and we strive to be around people most like ourselves to ensure this connection. You are taking steps to create cultural compatibility by hiring staff that share similar values. But try as you might for similarity, one organization's culture varies from the next, and your new staff members will need assistance in adapting to their new environment. They are in need of a personal network too, and will benefit from your cultural interpretation as they adapt!

> *Be nice, feel guilty and play safe. If there was ever a prescription for producing a dismal failure, that has to be it.*
>
> WALTER B. WRISTON

Q #14 How does gender as a culture reflect our diversity?

A Most of us understand the necessity today of avoiding cultural or racial bias and promoting cultural diversity. Often, however, one of the most confusing cultural issues, whether we are black, brown, white, born again New Age, agnostic, from the South, East, or Midwest, is our gender.

From the time when human beings were hunters and gatherers, there were distinctions between the sexes and their roles. (Most of us celebrate the physical differences!) There were hunters (mostly men) and gatherers (mostly women). In the fifties, when we were growing up, girls played dolls, house, and nurse, and boys played war. Even though we tried to raise our children without gender stereotype, our sons were fashioning guns out of their teething biscuits while they submerged their

Cabbage Patch dolls in the bathwater! Only within the last decade have we begun to research and understand our gender cultural diversity.

Neither male nor female tendencies are better or more correct, and all men and all women possess a mixture of each of these. Gender behavior may be influenced by past experiences, families of origin, and (as much as we may hate to admit that our rationality may be influenced by chemicals) hormones. Just as understanding each other's ethnic cultures allows us to work together more effectively, comprehension of gender characteristics allows us to communicate and relate with less confusion. Whenever males and females meet and communicate, be ready to identify the following characteristics that may be misunderstood.

- Males prefer independence; females prefer involvement. Females see connection and community as a source of power, while men, wanting to feel more independent, may make a decision without consultation. The need for consensus building may be more evident to females. (How many of you have we offended so far? Remember that all of us retain some male and some female characteristics, and that one way is not better than the other, merely different!) A common example is the tendency of some physicians (a larger percentage are male) to make decisions rather than undergo a group process for collaborating.

- Males prefer status to equality. Females tend to minimize differences and to use such words as "I don't know, what do you think?" to redress an imbalance of power in a conversation, thereby avoiding power inequities. Men are generally sizing up (and striving to the top of) the hierarchy in each situation and will therefore avoid hints and resist direction, but feel comfortable telling others what to do.

- While young females didn't learn to "win" and "lose" at dolls, young males learned to be criticized and to compete without carrying over negative feelings to their competitors. Females may wish to be helpful and cooperate, resisting conflict as a threat to connection. Males see conflict as necessary, a method of receiving status and power. As nurses, we see examples of this each day as many nurses (as females) tend to avoid conflict.

- Giving praise, information, and assistance with "fixing" things is a masculine trait, while some women will play the "poor little me" game and hope for rescue. (Thankfully, the "waiting to be a victim" role of women is assertively being stricken from the female repertoire. Unfortunately, we occasionally still see nurses asking physicians to fight battles for them with administration.)

- While a woman wishes to relate and communicate to establish rapport before getting to the "bottom line," men will want to do "report talk." "Decide what the problem is and fix it, and cut the extras," is often heard in meetings. Women must sometimes alter their excellent ability to establish rapport in order to cut to the main points of an argument to be heard. Men can adopt the more feminine rapport talk to establish common ground prior to negotiations or resolving conflict. Two books by Deborah Tannen (1986, 1990) elaborate on these traits.

- When listening, a man will generally refrain from giving gestures (such as nodding) unless he agrees with the point being made. A woman tends to nod, signaling listening, but may not agree with the speaker. These differences may be misinterpreted by the opposite gender, creating a misunderstanding. Consider the situation in which a female nurse has been talking with a male surgeon for several minutes about a patient situation. The surgeon walks away, having heard her, but doesn't acknowledge that he's received the message, leaving the nurse frustrated. Understanding the potential traits of the opposite sex, as well as your own, will enhance the health care team's ability to avoid relational ambiguity and to adapt to others' communication styles.

And that's the way it is.

WALTER CRONKITE

Q #15 I really want to be a good manager. But I feel so powerless when I have to deal with all these political issues. Can't we leave the politics out of it?

A Two major issues are at stake here: power and politics in the management setting. (Did you think your promotion just meant a day job with a title?) Many times we have heard a would-be manager state, "No thanks! I don't want to deal with the politics. It's not worth it!" In fact, our aversion to these issues is so great we've even heard nursing leaders proclaim that it is not possible to be political and professional at the same time. We would imagine that Florence Nightingale would take exception to this!

A little review of our history and the socialization process of women and men would probably enlighten us as to why these feelings are so strong. It's our guess that you male managers out there are probably skipping right over this question, while the female majority is rapidly reading on to see if we offer any quick remedies for this offensive aspect of the job. Let's take a look, with those of you that are still with us, at some of the background necessary for turning political know-how into a source of power in management.

- Understanding the definitions of each concept can remove some of the stigma surrounding these terms (which are not four letter words, by the way).
  Power: There are several definitions used to clarify this emotion loaded term. We suggest Webster's (1974, p. 544)

"authority—the ability to act or produce an effect"; or J.B. Miller's (1982) "the capacity to produce a change"; or Paul Hersey and Ken Blanchard's (1988) "the potential for influence." Sounds simple so far.

Politics: Again, we use Webster's (1974, p.537), "influencing or guiding governmental policy; competition between groups for power" or Diana Mason and Susan Talbott's (1985), "influencing the allocation of scarce resources."

Look at the terms used in these definitions. Influence, competition, change, authority. Terms that, as we were growing up, held very different meanings for us, depending on our gender. Think about the games you played as a child. Boys traditionally played team sports, learning to compete and to influence. Coaches held authority that was not questioned and changes in strategy were easily accepted. Girls played dolls and "house" for the most part, and learned to socialize and to keep the peace. The notion of winning and losing was not readily experienced and competition was not encouraged as girls focused on a sense of sharing and keeping things equal. (See Question 14 for a more complete review of gender.) Given this, it's a little easier to understand why a profession that is about 95 percent female feels uncomfortable with power and politics.

- Understand *your* feelings about politics and power. Looking at the definitions above and relating your childhood experiences, assess your comfort level. Nursing has often been criticized as a profession that is not organized and that has not maximized its full potential regarding the impact we could have on shaping health care policy, not to mention the policy and standards in our respective workplaces. Do you feel that any attempts to influence your leaders regarding your professional growth will be perceived as selfish? Do you hold back your ideas, not wanting to be perceived as power hungry? Or are you comfortable with the use of your expertise and do you communicate your ideas freely, while building relationships that will assist you strategically to improve your position?

Be aware that your staff, your followers, will be looking to you for an example. If you feel that you are powerless, that decisions are made that are out of your control, you will project this victimlike response to your staff as well. Assuming the victim role takes your and your unit out of the solution and only secures a powerless role of submission to the one that you grant power.

- Realize your sources of power and *use* them. Theory texts (this isn't one) generally list the sources of power as expert, information, referent, legitimate, reward, connection, and coercive. You may want to review one of the management texts for a refresher if these terms are not familiar to you.

- Develop both personal and position power. How many of you thought that this promotion, along with the new title and office, was your ticket to doing things *your* way? You may be able to influence the actions of the staff on your unit, because your position allows you hiring, evaluating, and firing ability. (The carrot and the stick approach.) This is position power, and as a new manager, is the most obvious and potentially most abused. Remember, this source of power was given to you, and can easily be taken away.

  Personal power is that which is developed by gaining the trust and confidence of those people on your team. Consistent performance, a caring attitude, being there at the tough times, all lead to the strengthening of these relationships. Having solutions, not complaints, helps to position you as a powerful person.

- Still not convinced that power and politics are important essentials in your position? Then consider your organization as a whole. Are you given a blank check for ordering supplies and hiring personnel? (We'd like to know who has found the horn of plenty!) If that is not the case, then you and the other units or departments are competing for a limited amount of resources. Influencing the decision makers boils down to politics, and how well you influence comes down to power. When the decision was made to order electronic thermometers, did they all go to the ICU while your unit was only allocated one (even though you have fifty two beds)? When a unit was selected for the new pilot project that results in an increase of the nurse–patient staffing ratio, was your unit the obvious choice? It was if you were visible, had built strong relationships with the decision makers, and presented a positive approach to the idea. *That's politics.*

- A final word about politics. The definitions and discussion above all relate to the idea of influence. And this influence is not limited solely to your unit within your organization. Continual professional development will take you into the arenas of your community, your professional organizations, and finally, the government, where the allocation of resources is decided daily. But that's another book! For now, just be aware that influencing decisions and selling your ideas is not limited solely to your working position.

> *One only receives that which is given. The game of life is a game of boomerangs. Our thoughts, deeds, and words return to us sooner or later, with astounding accuracy.*
>
> FLORENCE SCOVEL SHIN

Q #16 Why should I join a professional organization? And if it's so important, which one should I join?

A By the time you have taken on a management position, you are certainly aware of the many professional organizations that exist. If you were credentialed in a clinical specialty, such as critical care, you probably joined the local chapter of critical care nurses. The same is true for the operating room, the postanesthesia care unit, orthopedics, oncology, maternal–child health, and so on. In fact, we have often been criticized for having too many organizations. These splinter groups often serve to separate us rather than unite us in the one strong voice that would truly position our profession in a powerful role. We remember fondly one legislator from the Southwest complaining that there are too many "tribes" in nursing, and asking us to consider creating one group that could truly represent nursing. Wouldn't we love to do this! But, we digress . . . back to your questions.

- Check out the organization you are considering. We are reminded of a letter written long ago in which the nurse makes similar observations to those we commonly hear today. She wrote

  But concerning the deliberations of the "important meeting", they might just as well have been conducted in a foreign tongue so far as they held any significance for me. For what significance were, "desirable and well-educated applicants", "high standards for training schools", and "protection to the public" . . .

  This nurse made those remarks about a recent meeting she had attended of the Massachusetts State Nurses Association, held in 1915! Our point here is that until you allow yourself some time to get involved, and to network with some of the members, the first few meetings may seem like they are spoken in a foreign tongue. Before you are tempted to leave this foreign territory, ask some of the members what's going on. (If they don't know, that's a good sign you might want to move on out the door!)

- Look at the organization's membership, goals, and accomplishments. Who belongs to this group? Is it local and national, or a local specialty group that is not connected nationally? How are they perceived in the professional circle? Are members able to state their purpose, and are benefits as well as accomplishments visible? Be aware that every group will have some members who belong for unclear reasons, who do not actively participate, and may grumble that there is no point in belonging, but yet they write out that membership check annually. This raises another issue of importance: How much does it cost both in terms of time and money to belong?

- Determine what *you* want from being a member of this particular organization. Only you can decide what's in it for you. Don't overlook those intangible gains that professional membership can provide: the opportunity to network; the opportunity to better understand group process; a great arena for improving your leadership skills (many folks decide to go into management positions after being involved as a committee chair or an officer of the organization); visibility among your colleagues; the inside track on a new position that might be just right for you; mentorship by someone whom you admire and respect; and the chance to share ideas or problem solve similar experiences in practice. Let's not forget the obvious gains as well: representation on a national and local level so that as a profession we can be heard when policies are being shaped that affect nursing and health care; access to publications that will keep you current in new trends; access to research grants; reduced rates for credit cards (uh-oh! we're sounding like recruiters).

- Encourage professional development of your staff by sharing the information that you have gained. You may want to devote some time to each staff meeting for an organizational update, so that those who are members of various groups could share what's happening. If time is a factor at meetings, create a place on the unit where updates could be posted or shared, but at least take a moment to remind everyone that this information is available. Maybe a staff member would want to be the "organizational coordinator," keeping the unit current on organizational events, publications, and so on.

- By now you've probably guessed the answer to your second question. Deciding which organization to join is based on your personal needs. If you want exposure, visibility, and support in your new position, the local nursing management chapter of the American Organization of Nurse Executives would be a good choice. If staying connected with your specialty field is important, we recommend maintaining membership with that particular group as well. Once you've got your feet on the ground in your management position (it will happen!) and feel comfortable with your professional status, why not think about expanding your horizons? Membership in a professional business group, the local AIDS foundation, the Cancer Society, a church council, the school board, or the city council need the support and interest of us all. As health care managers, we would do well to consider stepping out of our defined role and lending our expertise to the community at large. Belong!

> *The world is full of willing people; some willing to work, the rest willing to let them.*

> ROBERT FROST

REFERENCES

"Concerning the Massachusetts State Nurses Association: A Change of Viewpoint." *The Massachusetts Nurse*, January 1993.

Hersey, P. & Blanchard, K. (1988). *Management of organizational behavior* (p.42). Englewood Cliffs, NJ: Prentice Hall, Inc.

Mason, D. & Talbott, S. (1985). *Political action handbook for nurses* (p. 29). Menlo Park, CA: Addison-Wesley Publishing Co., Inc.

Merriam-Webster Dictionary (1974). New York: Simon & Schuster.

Miller, J.B. (1982). *Colloquium: Women and power*. Wellesley College: Stone Center for Developmental and Service Studies.

Peters, T. (1987). Management by wandering around. In: Peters, Tom, ed. *Thriving on Chaos*. New York: Harper and Row, Perennial Library.

Tannen, D. (1986). *That's not what I meant*. New York: Ballantine Books.

Tannen, D. (1990). *You just don't understand*. New York: Ballantine Books.

CHAPTER 4

How Can I Put Together a Winning Team?

CREATION OF YOUR team is one of the most fundamental steps in making management work. Once you've selected the players, it's important to give them a sense of who they are (group identity) through stories and legends. Without developing trust in one another, they're unable to cooperate and work together to win. Understanding and developing comfort with their roles, whether they are catchers, pitchers, or playing right field, is essential for today's high performing health care team. Our answers to your questions about your team will help your clients to win as well!

> *Never doubt that a small group of thoughtful, committed people can change the world; indeed it is the only thing that ever has.*
>
> MARGARET MEAD

Q #17 I need help with selecting my team. Can I find out the truth if I'm not Barbara Walters? Can I stifle the urge to grovel and beg the candidate to take this job since it's a night position and we've been looking for years? Or do I use my cool, incisive, clinical questions to be certain this staff member isn't a sociopath in disguise?

A Interviewing, often regarded as a gamble at best, is a skill that may take years to perfect. But, even if you've interviewed enough candidates to people a small nation, there will be times that you choose the wrong person for the wrong job. Having begun with that disclaimer, you may think it's time to move on to the next question. However, as in any gamble, knowing what cards have been played before will assist you in making an intelligent decision.

- Recognize that an interview is designed for both of you. You wish to determine whether the candidate will fit in with your group and be able to do (or learn to do) the job, and the candidate is learning about you and your team and whether he or she would *want* to work with you.

- Use the interview as the beginning of an orientation. Share your group mission, vision, and some of the norms. Be honest. ("Yes, this department is known for being one of the most challenging, but we also have the best and most committed staff, and have had excellent quality data.")

- Be certain to find out about the positive and negatives of their past work experiences. Find out why they have chosen health care, what they like the most and the least. (If they hate paperwork and stress, and the job is rampant with both, it's best you both find out now.)

- If it becomes obvious early on in the interview that this candidate is not suitable for your department's needs, terminate the interview, keeping the following points in mind.

  □ As a representative of your organization, you will want to determine if there are other areas within the facility that may be a better fit.

  □ Make certain the interview is complete enough to project a positive image of your facility. Resist the temptation to end the interview too abruptly. "Don't let the door hit you on the way out" is not the politically correct phrase.

- Use situational questions that you have identified from experiences in your work area. "What would you do if a family member came to the department's desk, loudly stating that their loved one has received substandard care from your fellow staff?" "How would your coworkers describe you in a crisis situation?" Recalling situations that your department or you personally have had to deal with in the past can be a good source of situational examples. Real life situational questions are often the most indicative of the professional's ability to problem solve under pressure, and you'll sample their communication skills and delegation skills.

- If you are confused or concerned about salary, see our section on finance. End the interview on a positive note, with dignity and respect, but *never* promise a position, and *always* check references. Thank the person for his or her time and indicate some sort of time frame for follow-up.

- For the hiring decision: GO WITH YOUR GUT FEELING. Although we must always abide by fair hiring practices as well as union regulations and other organizational guidelines, remember that hiring mistakes will require an enormous amount of your time for follow-up, coaching, and possibly eventual termination. Waiting for another candidate is reasonable if you have serious concerns about the job fit after the first interview. Current trends point to the emergence of self-managing work teams, in which the team members are often involved in the interviewing process. Their intuition and gut feelings will help underscore the objective information you glean from discussion with the candidate. Just as experts advise against changing your first answer on an exam, there is no denying the power of your instinct.

- When you've gambled and lost, think about how you may have asked the right questions during the interview that would have alerted you to this person's problems. Keep each candidate's interview answers in a file, and review them after you've determined the job is a misfit. Look for any red flags that you might have missed that would have indicated that this person was not the best choice. But recognize that even Jimmy the Greek can't call all the odds correctly!

Let us train our minds to desire what the situation demands.

SENECA (4 B.C.–65 A.D.)

Q #18 So much depends on what the staff does. How can I trust them?

A "Trust your employees" is listed as the fourth key in James Autry's (1991) five guidelines for the manager in his book *Love and Profit*. And in a twenty page consultant report that came across our desk recently, the consultant cited the establishment of trust as a winning strategy for all CEOs. As important as it may seem, this elusive issue of trust is not given any in-depth attention in the standard management books. Is the concept an intuitive one, in which we all have a sense of the presence of trust? How then do we develop a confident reliance on the performance of a manager, fellow colleague, or employee?

Traveling the nation working with health care professionals to develop the skill of delegation, we have often faced this issue of trust. It is clearly not possible to give away a part of your job to someone else unless you trust in them, have faith on some level that they will not "mess up" or cause serious harm. Unless you are willing to work 24 hours a day doing the job yourself (You are? Then let us know—we're always looking for cheap labor—but can you be trusted?), you must become comfortable with developing a sense of trust.

1. Identify your predominant approach to trust. It should come as no surprise that researchers have found that humans tend to approach trust in one of two ways. (Those infamous researchers love to categorize behavior!) Basically, you are either a "giver" or a "withholder" when it comes to trust. The giver will freely extend trust to everyone, not taking it away unless proven wrong. The withholder will not grant his trust until it is earned. Your life experiences (how many times you've been burned, for instance) will determine your preferred practice in most relationships.

2. Understand how others handle trust. Just as we have predominant ways of extending or withholding trust, we tend to receive trust in one of two ways as well. Some individuals cannot accept trust. (This is a small group that you sometimes label as "can't be trusted" when, in fact, they are really individuals for whom we write the rules and watch carefully. These folks truly need and welcome controls and detailed rules.) The majority of us really thrive on trust, wanting the leeway to make our own choices and govern our own actions. (And no, we don't mean a rope to hang yourself on.) How do most members of your team respond?

3. Create an environment that says, "I trust you." (Here we are, asking you to work with the environment again. You'd think we expected you to be environmental specialists and not managers!) So much of what we do in management works against a positive environment. Think about it. How do your personnel policies read? How do you handle absences? We bet you have some method of tracking the number of times an employee is absent, so that you can monitor potential abuse. What does this say about trust? Many times we act as police

rather than as managers of adults who are working together to achieve a common goal.

4. Define your behavior regarding trust. As discussed above, there are many situations in which you are placed in the position of monitor. When the rules are written and enforced in such a manner that says daily, "We don't really trust you," it's difficult to overcome that perception and foster creative development in your employees. How much attention you pay to the regulatory details will tell your staff members in a big way how you really feel about trusting them. We worked with one hospital that had a tremendous morale problem that was improved by rewriting the dress code. Instead of four pages addressing everything from nail polish to chewing gum, we encouraged management to let the staff create their own code. (Getting management to agree to this was about as easy as pushing a truck through the eye of a needle, but that's what we get paid for!) The dress code the staff wrote was one paragraph, speaking to the rights of patients and employees alike to expect health care workers to dress professionally and act accordingly. It was beautiful!

Those who trust us, educate us.

George Eliot

Q #19 When something goes wrong, I take all the blame. Can't I take the credit too?

A We all remember playing the childhood game, follow the leader. The rules are very simple: Pick one person to be the leader and everyone else to do exactly what the leader does. For most of industrial history, this has been the traditional story of management. In today's world, we are beginning to focus on group theory and self managed teams.

Nevertheless, there will still be a distinction, although not as sharp, between the leadership and the followers of the group. As children, we may not have been quite sure of the point of the game, but we always knew we wanted to be the leaders. Being the leader looked like a lot more fun; being in the spotlight and getting to decide what to do was more rewarding than doing what you were told. But our friends didn't all feel that way, and many were comfortable *not* being the leader. (Thank goodness, for what's a leader without someone to follow?)

Looking back, we realize that the success of that children's game depended a great deal on how well the followers cooperated. Usually the game ended when the leader's actions became too complicated or the followers became bored with the leader and broke into disorganized gales of laughter. (Aren't you sometimes tempted to do that now?)

In today's management game, even though we intend to move in a *team* direction, we continue to give star billing and major attention to the leader. Leadership development seminars abound, textbooks are filled with defining leaders and effectively improving their skills. Unfortunately, little attention has been paid to the very important role of the follower. And yet, the success of any unit, be it a business, a hospital department, or a professional organization, is dependent to a great degree on the performance of the followers, those unsung heroes who are essential to the achievement of the leader's vision.

In reaching for the professional growth health care hopes to achieve in the years ahead, cooperative effort and creative participation will be the pathway to success. We must realize that the successful follower will not necessarily mimic the leader but will display individual creative thought and action in harmony with the mission of the group. How can this be achieved?

• Recognize the importance of the "followership" role. Typically, the leader is in the spotlight, and the actions of the supporting players are overlooked. If this happens too often in your group, you may find the game disintegrating no matter how clever the leader is. When the board of directors praises you, as the critical care manager, for the wonderful new open heart protocol, do you share this acclaim with the staff? (Or privately savor the moment, knowing it was your willingness to take the initiative and organize the staff members to write the protocol *they* suggested?)

- Identify the performance expectations of the follower. It is impossible to achieve a goal unless the objectives are clearly identified. Followership frustration results when communication from the leader is lacking or unclear. Remember the game of follow the leader and how frustrated you were when everyone just stood there or did something completely different from what you wanted? Making the expectations clear is primarily the leader's responsibility and will help the team to follow your lead. Set aside time weekly to meet with individuals on your staff and check with them about current operations, plans for changing documentation, and their perceptions of how things are going.

- Foster independent, creative thinking. The objectives you've established may no doubt be attained in several different ways. Encouraging followers to choose their own path stimulates cooperation and creative energy. Positive support, not criticism, of independent choices develops accountability and increases self-confidence. When someone proposes a new way of handling the accounts in outpatient care, how do you respond? Do you give the person your attention and discuss the idea or brush it off as not important right now? And further, if the idea doesn't work as well as everyone hopes, how is this handled? Fear of negative consequences will stifle any creativity you may hope to foster.

I can easier teach twenty what were good to be done, than be one of the twenty to follow mine own teaching.

WILLIAM SHAKESPEARE

Q #20 I've been hearing lots of stories since I took this job. Should I pay attention? Do group legends and stories have a place in my department?

A Each work group, each unit, each department must share its precious group legends to pass along a sense of "who we are." The values of the team are thereby enjoyed and relived as the stories are repeated for the pleasure of the elders and for the edification of the initiates. There is real magic in recalling and sharing fantastic achievements, hilarious events, and examples of individuals who have performed beyond the norm but who exemplify the best qualities of the team. Remember, some exaggeration sweetens the experience! Some may be unforgettable events, some may seem insignificant, but all are important records of your group's evolution.

• Overcoming the impossible using humor—"The Case of the Exploding Toilet"

During a construction project, the plumbing system at a large tertiary care center went awry. As the nurses completed charting near the cardiac monitors on this step-down cardiac care unit, a huge rush of water, as wide as the door and knee-high, whooshed out of a patient's room. Riding the wave was a still-full urinal. Amazed and dismayed, one of the nurses exclaimed, "I thought that dosage of diuretic was too high!" While the waters continued to flow, the nursing and environmental services departments coped extremely well to avoid injury to patients with pacers (bedridden and

*connected to electrical machinery) and narrowly avoided a
total shutdown of the medical center's main computer. They
sang of their "Code Noah" in tune with some old Northwest
sailing jigs.*

Team values expressed: Bring on *any* disaster, we can cope!
And keep our sense of humor!

- Individuals who exemplify our spirit—"Nancy and the Thunderbird Wine"

*On the medical unit in a large community hospital, many of
the visitors brought extra special get well gifts, sometimes
inclusive of illicit drugs and liquor. Early on one of her first
shifts as a new graduate, two burly, reeling gentlemen
wished to visit Nancy's patient. Soon after they entered the
room, there was a crash, and we smelled a noxious bouquet
wafting down the hall. Nancy strode purposefully from the
room with the remaining Thunderbird wine under her arm,
stating, "I am pouring out this wine! I have notified our
visitors that this is unacceptable behavior and will only
serve to harm their friend in his present condition." The
men were ushered meekly away by security guards.*

Team values expressed: We have courage and self-confidence, and we aren't afraid to deal with the "seamier" sides
of life.

- Stories of our leaders—"Of Lice and Leadership"

*Crowd control was the problem, when friends of our lice-
ridden patients visited and deposited more of the parasites
on the respiratory unit. Housekeeping had vacuumed a
snowy drift of the dead creatures from the lounge chairs.
While using the phone, the nurse manager saw lice on her
desk mess, each lively creature salivating at the thought of
making her hair his new mobile home! The manager, being
new, panicked. After all, it was like an invasion, with pri-*

vate territory under siege! Now at anxiety level four, the nurse manager forgot about keeping the narcotics available, how to use the phone, and other necessary details while the area was taped closed and fogged with insecticide. As a result, everyone on the unit was in an uproar and barely able to complete everyday tasks. The next day, she recognized that, as leader, losing her cool adversely affected everyone on the unit. She apologized to all the staff, who appreciated the honesty and laughed about the incident for years. "Remember the lesson of the louse!"

Team values expressed: We recognize that our behavior as leaders affects our patients and those with whom we work. We respect people who admit when they're wrong, and we'll forgive them.

- Short and fun stories—"The Dress Code"

  All departments noted that the dress code for physicians at a certain time in history consisted of white shoes and a white belt. For some of the younger set, jeans became the casual and more comfortable alternative. One Saturday, a physician who never wore anything but a three-piece-suit wore jeans. They were designer jeans, and pressed, but they were jeans. The staff noted this day on their calendar and celebrated it each year with a "Best Dressed Contest."

Team value expressed: We enjoy noticing the idiosyncrasies of those with whom we work. We will celebrate *anything!*

- Fantastic achievements as a group

  Think about difficult situations within your department, whether they be patient-oriented or not, and some of the great successes you have had by pulling together with other groups. Fill in the distinguishing characteristics, and you've got a great start at recording your own legends.

☐ Get together with staff members and talk about some of the most precious, funny, exciting moments they've had working in your department. Be certain to include those veterans as well as the novices.

☐ Make a list of some of the most important events. Ask someone to be the group historian and keep track of important stories in a special journal in your department. Some of these may be permanently in print if you use a department newsletter format as part of your internal marketing.

☐ At parties or other social events, listen for stories and ask people to write them down or put them on audiotape.

☐ Use the stories to illustrate points in team meetings or when orienting new people. Be certain that all staff members recognize the value of their rich heritage, and encourage them to prize new events, passing on their knowledge to new employees.

Every family, every college, every corporation, every institution need tribal storytellers. The penalty for failing to listen is to lose one's history, one's historical context, one's binding values. . . . Without the continuity brought on by custom, any group of people will begin to forget who they are.

MAX DEPREE

Q #21 Someone from the night shift told the supervisor that the staff from the "off shifts" don't even recognize my face! A 24-hour work day doesn't sound like fun to me! How can I be expected to attend all these meetings from 7:00 A.M. to 6:00 P.M. as well as interact with each shift?

A   You've probably worked your share of "off shifts" in the past and you may be wondering *why* your staff can't understand your managerial obligations during the daytime, weekday hours. Working with your staff from other shifts may be difficult due to such logistical challenges as child-care coverage, classes, or other responsibilities. Maybe your body rebelled against working evenings or nights in the past, and you found yourself desperate for sleep at 4:00 A.M. despite consuming 12 cups of espresso. However, regardless of the time management problems inherent in maintaining contact with all your staff, you've been hired for twenty-four-hour management responsibility. It's essential that these people not only read your name from your name badge, but know *who* you are as a person and as a leader.

• Review your calendar and plot times for contact with other shifts. Come in early one day each week to interact with those on the overnight shift. Plan to stay late to talk with those on the afternoon and evening shifts. If you have difficulty doing this, plan as far ahead as necessary. Come in late if you're leaving late; set up breakfast with a friend so that you give yourself extra motivation for sticking to the plan. Make that appointment with the hairdresser for the days you come in early so that you'll have to leave on time.

• In your yearly planning, find at least one holiday on which you'll visit your staff and bring goodies. This will help staff understand that you *are* thinking of them while you enjoy your time with family and friends. Some managers work holidays from time to time to keep in touch with how systems function. This is a great suggestion. However, don't become a martyr either.

• Weekends can be considered another "off shift," especially if you employ a "weekend only" staff. These employees are isolated from the usual communication channels and may not have a clear understanding of the department's mission and vision. They'll benefit from your presence.

- Maintain close contact with the house supervisors, if you are lucky enough to have them. Ask them how they think things are going in your department during their tours of duty. They'll have excellent suggestions for development of some staff members and many positive messages about others.

- When you are at work during hours other than the daytime, be certain you are visible. Make rounds; spend time with your office door open. This is a great time to inform those on the alternate shifts about "nice to know" issues. For example, let them know how things are shaping up with pet projects; what's happening with the organization's strategic plan; that you are aware of their concerns. It's also an opportunity to let them know what you've been doing so your role is clarified in their minds. They'll worry less about how frequently they see your face when they know you're representing their interests while they sleep.

- Plan staff meetings so that all the personnel from each shift are available to attend. This may mean repeating the meetings several times throughout the day and evening. Some organizations record staff meetings on tape (audio or video) in addition to written minutes. Although many facilities attempt to keep staff meeting salary expenses and overtime to a minimum, there is great danger in staff missing necessary face-to-face discussion with the manager and other members of the team. When staff don't understand the direction they are supposed to be going, nor have time to discuss their specific obstacles or concerns, you can expect additional conflict and quality problems.

- Attend shift parties or functions when asked. (We hope they'll want you to be there!) These activities are a wonderful opportunity to get to know your staff as people, and you'll certainly hear about the challenges they face on their shifts.

- Keep track of attendance at staff meetings and inservices. Which staff are not maintaining contact with the organization? Invite them, include them. Let them know their input is valuable. If they continue to resist involvement, let them know your expectations. (Check the job descriptions also; is attendance and involvement included? If not, you may wish to add some performance standards that would reflect your reasonable expectations.)

- Involve employees from all shifts in group task forces and committees. Let them know you respect their unique perspectives.

- At least once a year, spend time individually with each staff member. If you are also their immediate supervisor, you'll want to increase the frequency. (See Question 25 on performance evaluation.) Thank them for their hard work. Ask them how they are doing professionally and how they evaluate the department's strengths and weaknesses. This should be a meeting emphasizing positive planning and mentoring. You'll also discover any pressing concerns while you are enjoying time with each staff member.

- Remember that despite overwhelming schedules, your visibility is as essential to promoting your vision as light is to the proper functioning of the eye.

> *The great leader is not the one in the spotlight, he or she's the one leading the applause.*
>
> ANONYMOUS

Q #22 Sometimes it seems like it's "nursing against the world." I know other departments dislike nursing because we complain and expect a lot. How can we work together more effectively as an interdisciplinary team?

A Occasionally we find ourselves wanting to hold onto the status quo of traditional turf. In nursing departments across the country, we are just awakening to our powerful, central position in directing the care of the patients and systems of health care organizations. Because we have just begun to enjoy our positions of power, it's tough for us to realize that we must work together collaboratively with all of the disciplines and supporting services to make certain we keep pace with the changes of the nineties. Those organizations that remain fixed into set boundaries ("You deliver the medications, she cleans the room, and I do the nursing care as I define it, and let's not discuss it further!") will perish, squeezed in the vise of cost containment and quality imperatives.

How can you and your staff develop useful, cooperative relationships with all the other workers who support you and work with our patients? We've spent many hours of continuing education schooling ourselves and our staff members to overcome prejudice against other colors, cultures, genders, and those who are disabled. We use the same process to "unlearn" the professional prejudices we've picked up since our student days.

1. Identify your own group characteristics. How do you see yourselves? How do other departments see you? (Are nurses considered assertive within your own unit, while the pharmacists consider you pushy or downright aggressive when the medications aren't up on time?) Try to understand how you may seem to others. This step helps you open up your minds to possible self-induced discrimination.

2. Define your strengths as a department. What are your most important goals? (For nursing, quality patient care will most likely be number one.) What are the goals of the

other departments? (Environmental services' main objective may be to provide a spotless environment.)

3. List common goals among departments and professions. We suspect that all will contribute to quality patient care, but it's important that nurses understand that other groups may have a different approach to achieving the same end result.

4. Identify the stereotypes you may hold of other groups or professions. (Do you see the physicians as generally being self-centered bullies? Do you think social workers are usually more interested in the processing of information than in action? Are these beliefs factual?) Examining stereotypes and how you developed them will open eyes to the barriers we generate internally. They may have had some basis in factual observation in one case, but these generalizations will inhibit us from working together toward common goals. The common goal again? Yes, we need to understand each other to work together more effectively for quality patient care!

5. Discuss what drives you crazy about members of other groups or professions. You may find the words "back-ordered," or "we're busy too," or "can't you take care of this type of patient on *your* unit?" to be a call to arms. Identify those trigger words that cause you to lose perspective. Then, when you hear them, take time out to bring yourself back to rationality before reacting.

6. List the "alert words" that, when verbalized, will alert you to the possibility of professional discrimination brewing. These may be such words as always, never, we, they, and other generalizations. For example, "Intensive care *always* forgets to get the med reordering done!" "Surgery *never* remembers to record the final vital signs before transfer." "*They* are just like that, *they* don't care." "*We* always do a better job with infectious disease pa-

tients." "You can't count on the transporters around here."

7. Recognize patterns or frequency of communication. Have you stopped talking at all to the maintenance department unless there's an emergency? If so, barriers have been built. As a manager, you must identify the priority groups who have been given the silent treatment. (These groups are probably also being described with the "alert words.") Understanding the barriers allows you to lead your staff members to be first to break down those walls. Let them know you believe, "It's time to understand each other better as a group and as individuals to improve the efficiency and effectiveness of all our efforts!"

8. Begin to understand (and talk about) the strengths of the other professions or departments. They have specific skills and perspectives that nursing lacks. (Yes, it's hard to imagine, but another group may truly have valuable input into the care of our patients!) For example, it probably *does* help patient care if the pharmacy is very careful and deliberate in getting the orders filled. The admitting department isn't singling out your unit for punishment with so many admissions, but they *are* concerned that the patients get immediate care instead of languishing on a gurney in the emergency department. (For more in-depth discussion of some of these points, an excellent reference is Peg Neuhauser's *Tribal Warfare in Organizations.)*

9. Celebrate the impact of those perspectives and different skills and traits on the group's common goal of quality patient care. Nursing cannot do it alone; nor should we want to! Our patient care team must include all of the people that work with us and those that we may not see, but that support us and our patients.

10. Make it a policy to develop intragroup trust by reinforcing the expectation that all people, internal and external to your organization, must be *consistently* treated with respect, care, encouragement, and concern.

Diversity: The art of thinking independently together.

MALCOLM FORBES

Q #23 I have to let someone go and I feel awful about it. Is it possible to terminate someone without trauma?

A Which dictator was it that believed that firing a subordinate meant the firing squad? If so, it's unfortunate we use the word "fire" to mean termination of someone's employment with us.

None of us likes to fail at anything. But trying to perform a job that isn't right for us isn't failing, it's like the proverbial "fitting a square peg into a round hole." It's uncomfortable for the peg and disfigures the hole.

1. If it's obvious that a staff member is not going to be able to fit in or do the job appropriately, it's time to think about what other roles may match the employee's strengths and preferences. Since all staff members are potentially valuable somewhere in the organization, find out what other positions may interest this person. Human beings are our most valuable resource; try to salvage this person for your organization if he or she is a good organizational culture/values match.

2. New employees must be given written standards and performance expectations. During the first months of employment, they must be given direct and clear feedback about how their performance measures up. Also, explore how they feel about the job and how things are going for them.

3. If problems occur, be clear about which performance objectives are below standard. Help them understand how to improve, and ask them to fashion an improvement plan with a timeline. Some people don't know where to start on this, and you may need to give them examples and enlist the assistance of a clinical educator.

4. In today's litigious society, documentation is essential. In most cases, verbal discussion is followed by written documentation of what objective events or actions do not meet the performance expectations, what you jointly agree upon for a plan, and when you'll meet again to discuss progress. Depending on your facility's policies as well as union contracts, two or more counseling sessions and documents may have to be completed before termination seems appropriate. This will depend on the gravity of the employee's offenses. Consult with your human resources department if you are inexperienced in this.

5. Always approach your discussions in the spirit of coaching (see Question 27). Following someone around to prove they should be let go is beneath the dignity of the manager and the employee, reflecting a nasty, adversarial management image to all employees.

6. If there is no job fit, it's better to help the employee recognize this and encourage him or her to move on to a different role. Generally, asking the employee if he or she is happy in the job will begin a discussion of what type of position would be better suited to his or her preferences and strengths. Whether it's uncomfortable to terminate the employee or not, if you don't bother to deal with the problem and encourage the employee to move on, your good performers will move on themselves!

7. Strive to communicate honestly and directly, giving positive as well as the necessary negative feedback to the employee, so that he or she will welcome the change to a

more appropriate role. Many (not all) of those we have terminated have thanked us for helping them see that they were unhappy and needed a better fit!

Dobkins, I just don't know WHAT we're going to do without you. But we're going to try.

DAVID FROST

(from "The Sack and How to Give It.")

REFERENCES

Autry, J. (1991). *Love and profit: The art of caring leadership.* New York: William Morrow & Co.

Neuhauser, P. (1988). *Tribal warfare in organizations.* New York: Ballinger Publishers.

CHAPTER 5

___

How Can I Work Team Magic
with Motivation?

WHAT KIND OF magic is required to encourage people to work together smoothly, at their top performance level, even with enthusiasm, under extremely challenging circumstances?

Your boss may have encouraged you to improve your style of "motivating your people," as if you had not yet located the mysterious key to management Nirvana. In this chapter, we'll open the door and examine some pathways that lead to an energized, empowered staff. First we'll look at our own motivation, to gain a primary understanding of how this psychological principle works. Performance evaluation and coaching can be used as motivational tools, but the methods used are important to the final result. We all nod in agreement that we should empower ourselves and our staff, but what does this mean in terms of managerial behavior on a daily basis?

It's true that we, as managers, can't *make* another person motivated. Motivation comes from within the individual. But we are accountable for creating an environment that encourages us all to reach beyond our perceived potential.

> *Oh heavens, how I long for a little ordinary human enthusiasm. Just enthusiasm—that's all. I want to hear a warm, thrilling voice cry out Hallelujah! Hallelujah! I'm alive!*

> JOHN OSBORNE

Q #24 What's my role in motivating the staff? How can I make them want to do what I say?

A There are many motivational theories that we could refer you to, from Maslow (Question 34) to McGregor's theory X and theory Y to Herzberg's theory of motivation and hygiene. No matter what theory you study and apply, the basic idea remains the same. You *cannot* motivate people. (No, we're not going to let you off the hook that easily!) As a manager, you set the stage and facilitate the environment so that the individual is self-motivated to respond in the way that meets his or her needs and the needs of the unit. What do we mean by that? Let's see.

- Look at the approach you take toward your employees. Is it as positive as it could be, or do you rule with the idea that no one can be trusted and constantly remind staff of their shortfalls and mistakes? Or do you approach staff members and the unit as a whole with the idea that they are winners, doing a good job overall, supported and valued by you and the organization? This will make all the difference in how willingly your staff pulls together and works to make the unit a success. You *can* control your approach.

- A positive comment, a thank-you, a raise, an increase in authority through delegation can all play an important part in establishing an environment where people feel appreciated. Think about it. Psychology teaches us about the self-fulfilling concept: As a person thinks, so shall he become. If the staff see themselves as highly regarded and valued employees, they will go a long way to continue this feeling. Conversely, if they feel that what they do doesn't count, they will continue to be marginal performers. We like the list of questions posed by Max DePree (1989) in his book *Leadership Is An Art*. In it he states that the working environment can be looked at in a variety of ways by asking these questions:

☐ Does what I do count?

☐ Does what I do make a difference to anybody?

☐ Why should I come here?

☐ Can I be somebody here?

☐ Is there *for me* any rhyme or reason here?

☐ Is this a place where I can learn something?

☐ Would I show this place to my family—or am I ashamed to show it to them—or does it just not matter?

We suggest using these questions as your own personal inventory for both your motivation and position satisfaction as well as that of your staff. Perhaps sharing this list with staff would be a good place to start taking a "wellness check" of your unit.

• What does your rule book look like? Are your policies strict and punitive? We tend to write rules for the small minority who have a tendency to be out of line. Unfortunately, this sends a message to the rest of the staff that is demoralizing and demotivating. How you emphasize and enforce these policies will either reinforce that lack of trust or will let people know that you are a fair player who is more interested in positive development than negative punishment. (Are you requiring a doctor's excuse for every sick call? We're sure the physicians appreciate the business, but what's the message?)

• How do you deal with mistakes? Because so much is at stake when we care for our patients, we have adopted a rather punitive way of looking at mistakes. Think of the language we use: "She *committed* a med error." This makes it sound like she is guilty of the most serious offense and must be punished accordingly. How do we learn in an environment like this? And more importantly, is anyone going to be willing to do anything differently, to take a risk with a new idea, if the chances for ridicule and punishment are that great? We're not saying that the issue of medicine errors is not serious. Far from it. But if your approach is 1–2–3 strikes, you're out, then be prepared for reluctant staff members who will be locked into maintaining the status quo, will resist your new ideas, and will certainly not put forth any of their own.

- Tune in to the radio station WIIFM. We all listen to it, including your staff. "What's In It For Me?" is one of the first questions we are likely to ask when faced with a new opportunity or suggestion. It may sound selfish, but we all like to feel that there will be some personal benefit to the action we are being asked to take. Be prepared to have a few ideas in response, or better yet, have your staff members answer what they'd like to see in it for themselves. Careful! They may just tell you!

Good and evil, reward and punishment, are the only motives to a rational creature: these are the spurs and reins whereby all mankind are set on work, and guided.

JOHN LOCKE

Q #25 I don't feel comfortable being the judge and the jury on my unit. How can I make performance evaluations positive for me and for my staff?

A Are your performance reviews often late? Are they molding on the bottom of the pile on your desk as one of your most distasteful tasks? When you call an employee into your office for his or her evaluation meeting, do you hear other staff groan, "Now you're in for it!"? If any of these apply to you, it's time for a change!

We all remember the purposes of performance evaluations: to provide feedback to the employee; to validate movement to another pay level; to fulfill the Joint Commission on Accreditation of Healthcare Organizations (Joint Commission) or other policy requirements. In the current fast-paced, team-oriented, quality-driven health care environment, there is no room for activities that have not been designed to ensure your organization's ability to adapt and respond resiliently to that environment. How can we redesign performance evaluation to promote the necessary attributes of the health care worker of the twenty first century?

- Rethink your objectives for performance review. The time you take to meet personally with an employee can be fruitful for accomplishment of interacting goals.

  □ providing positive feedback about the employee's most positive contributions to the team efforts

  □ mentoring staff members for future career opportunities

  □ obtaining feedback about your organization's strengths and weaknesses—what is going well and what is not

  □ gathering creative ideas for cost-effectiveness, change

  □ receiving feedback on your own leadership and managerial skills

  □ re-establishing common goals

- Evaluate your performance review forms with a jaundiced eye. The form should reflect the true values and mission of the organization. Objective, measurable performance criteria should be used. Is it possible to use the form for keeping official track of the employee's goals and how they will contribute to team objectives? Are educational needs easily retrievable for planning? Can information be easily placed into a file in your personal computer?

- If you have never done performance reviews before, consult with your human resources department for suggestions. Just as in interviewing, you must steer clear of personal topics (unless the employee is asking for assistance) and discuss measurable, objective behaviors. If you are planning any disciplinary measures, discuss your documentation with your personnel advisors.

- Although your personnel policies may require a yearly official review, once per year is not enough feedback in this changing world. Interim meetings are necessary quarterly or more frequently. Keeping notes of discussions in an informal way will help keep the manager and the employees on track for mutual goals.

- If you aren't aware of the Joint Commission's requirements for performance evaluation, consult their most recent standards. Yearly competencies reviews and skill checklists will be an essential portion of your evaluation process.

- Since we are in a service business, it is helpful to include feedback from clients, co-workers, and other departments. How well does this person communicate with the various internal and external publics? This is an essential topic for discussion and coaching (see Question 27).

- Prior to meeting with employees, ask them to complete their own reviews. Ask them:

    ☐ What do you want to accomplish in the following year, and in the next three years?

    ☐ What problems do you see as the most pressing at this time?

    ☐ What concerns have you had about your performance?

    ☐ Do you see signs of impending challenges, and what should we do about them now?

☐ What am I doing that helps you and impedes you, and how can I, as your manager, better help you grow?

• Avoid the "halo or horn" syndromes. If some of your staff can do no wrong, but some seem to be poor in all areas, re-evaluate your objectivity. Each employee has strengths and weaknesses. Your star performers may seem perfect in every way, but they must be aware of their own need to grow in certain performance objectives. Those who seem to be wallowing in an uncertain job match still possess some strengths that they contribute to the team effort. If you can't uncover *any* strengths, you should have already consulted our answers for termination without trauma.

• Think of performance reviews as private forums with employees, giving both of you an opportunity to identify learning needs, celebrate successes, generate creative ideas to solve problems, and reaffirm mutual direction toward organizational goals.

> *Only children and immature adults believe that life is a contest of strength, a win-or-lose situation. The battleground of health care management is strewn with the cadavers of managers who constantly practiced adversarial techniques to obtain cooperation. One does not mandate cooperation by punishing, threatening, or by legislating.*
>
> LAWRENCE C. BASSETT AND NORMAN METZGER

Q #26 People keep talking about empowerment. Isn't this just participative management? Or do I really need to make this happen in my department?

A Whether your organization is implementing the principles of quality management in terms of continuous quality improvement (CQI) or total quality management (TQM), empowered interdisciplinary teams are essential ingredients in reaching beyond a minimum level of service quality. Empowering means that the members of the team have been given the authority, responsibility, and accountability for the product or service they produce. Beyond participative management, these individuals feel they are able to go beyond "giving input" and are encouraged to be creative, to think and dream, to direct the progress of the organization by their efforts. They feel ownership in outcomes, take initiative, are encouraged to grow, and enjoy the work itself. As you can see, empowerment moves beyond the concept of asking your staff to give input to decisions you're probably going to make yourself anyway (participative management as it is often practiced).

To illustrate a fundamental point about empowerment, Mike, an investigative reporter of the Middle Ages, was interviewing two stone cutters at a quarry in Italy. Mike asked the first about his job. He replied, "It's horrible; these substandard tools are never available on time, it seems like slavery, all I do is make square blocks of stone!" Mike moved on to the other stone cutter and asked him to take some time to discuss his job with him. He replied, "I don't have much time to talk with you, and please keep your distance! You see, I am creating a cathedral!"

- The first most essential step in empowering your staff (and yourself) is to provide a clear sense of purpose. The second stone cutter knew the end result he was shooting for and the importance of his work in the creation of a magnificent house of worship.

- Empowerment includes encouraging the individual to take on increasing responsibility commensurate with his or her strengths, and providing the needed education to fill in the gaps.

- Empowerment includes investing in training again and again. This education must include skills in communicating with others effectively, conflict resolution, and overcoming professional turf battles as well.

- Information is a basis of power. Staff members should be aware of all that is going on administratively and be involved in the long-term planning. Withholding information (often so that staff members aren't "upset") is paternalistic and will destroy the trust that has been gained.

- Encourage your team to be creative, innovate, take risks. In health care, we have often avoided risks because of the patients that could be harmed. Obviously, it's essential not to take risks with patients! However, this has been one of the many excuses we have used in health care to move more slowly than any other public sector in adapting to change.

- Innovative individuals and teams must feel free to make mistakes, try new things, and learn from them. Blame must be removed from our management vocabulary. (Dangerous clinical errors obviously must be dealt with aggressively. Here we are speaking of new ideas, systems revamping, integrative forecasting, and the like.)

- As manager, listen, listen, and listen again. Be certain that group problem-solving efforts meet with real improvements.

- Provide resources to the team! As a manager, you have moved away from a command and control method of leadership to a coaching, encouraging, and facilitating mode. Remove the barriers that keep your group from moving ahead.

- Be flexible and adaptable to change. It is the *avoiding* of change that causes the pain.

  Powerlessness corrupts. Absolute powerlessness corrupts absolutely.

  ROSABETH MOSS KANTER

Q #27 I've heard that I'm not supposed to be a manager anymore. I'm supposed to be a coach. I've never been fond of sports, so please explain: How can I become a winning coach?

A It sometimes seems a lot easier just to *tell* people what to do, rather than participating in the painstaking process of mentoring, facilitating, teaching, and encouraging them to grow and mature in their roles. Some staff members are easy to coach; others more challenging. (This is an understatement of reality in many cases.) As self-managing work teams develop, and as more and more of the middle management are "downsized" out of jobs, many managers find it difficult to resist the seductive urge to keep teams dependent on their leadership, thereby building evidence for a continued paycheck. Health care managers must find methods to resist the "empty nest" syndrome and begin to conceptualize their jobs differently.

We've evolved beyond paternalistic/maternalistic, command and control management styles into what is often called "coaching." When using this term, remove the images of the abusive, screeching football coach who spends hours detailing the errors from each game. Instead, think of the positive leaders who encourage all of the players to excel through their specific use of visual and verbal communications.

• Repeat constantly the vision and mission of your organization. (We do not mean to repeat this in the form of a mantra. Instead, find ways to weave your constants into your conversations, meetings, problem solving, report times.) Each member of the team must know how his or her performance is essential to achieve your team goals. ("Your interaction with that family was wonderful. Certainly they must have known that quality patient care comes first around here!")

- Use specific examples of positive results. "Our home health organization provides the most comprehensive, cost-effective, responsive care possible to every client in our community." "Our interdisciplinary team has been judged AAA⁺ quality by our patients who have had coronary artery bypass grafts. We have also cut two days and $200,000 from the budget for each patient." "Our pharmacy is the best, and excels in providing self-medication training. Our clients receive the highest quality professional care in the community." Don't limit this praise to verbal exchanges—put it in writing; use symbols. (See celebrating success, Question 28.)

- Give recognition for ideas. Most of us recall a situation, very demotivating, when we expressed a great idea, and our manager took total credit for it.

- Coaching means giving positive and negative feedback. The value of giving specific, honest, positive feedback as often as possible can't be overstated. "John, I saw how well you handled that complaint. You certainly handled them calmly, but showed you cared. Your follow-through was excellent. We could have lost a whole family, but you'll keep our organization busy with returning clients!"

- Giving negative feedback is often very difficult. If you'll follow the following recipe, the process will be much less threatening to both you and your staff member.

  1. Give the employee credit for all his or her efforts. Recognize positive contributions.

  2. Ask for feedback regarding the specific situation. Often, things are not as they first seem. Enter the discussion in a teaching frame of mind: Adult learners must know the importance and relevance of the topic.

  3. Give feedback on your impressions or concerns about the problem. Be specific.

4. Discuss when there are gaps between your expectations and what really happened. Explore what each of you would expect to happen differently in the future.

5. Ask the employee for ideas on how the problem can be avoided. Be ready to give assistance if this is an educational problem, or if you need to be involved in systems adjustments or problem solving.

6. Discuss the employee's plan and set another time for discussing progress.

7. Give the employee immediate feedback when you see improvements or if the plan is not working as you expected.

- One of the most often neglected coaching skills is helping work teams clearly develop the following details:

  ☐ a goal that causes some stretching but is not totally unrealistic

  ☐ the outcomes needed from the project

  ☐ how to measure progress or lack of it

  New self-managing teams often spend weeks wallowing in the details of these issues. The manager's experience is invaluable in helping design a clear course. Just remember the questions our children often ask on car trips: "Where are we going?" "How long will it take to get there?" "How will we know we are getting close?" "Are we there yet?"

- Whenever possible, the members of the team should be able to develop methods of self-monitoring and giving themselves feedback on their progress. This is exceptionally motivating, but doesn't replace your role as coach to:

  ☐ Encourage

  ☐ Praise

☐ Give feedback

☐ Remove barriers

☐ Provide resources

☐ Celebrate success!

> *One man may hit the mark, another blunder; but heed not these distinctions. Only from the alliance of the one, working through and with the other, are great things born.*
>
> SAINT-EXUPERY

Q #28 You keep talking about celebrating success. Health care is serious business. Is it really important to celebrate?

A How can we celebrate when we deal with pain and suffering and death and illness? But these are all realities of life and, as health care professionals, we know what to do to help our fellow human beings get through these tragedies. We can commend ourselves for using our skills to cure, to support, to help. And we can revel in the joys in health care: a patient saved, the birth of a long awaited child, the relief of pain, the prevention of disease, the camaraderie of teamwork.

What is life, if it's not to be enjoyed? If you or your team members don't find some joy in your work, then it's time to find other jobs or professions. Human beings derive some satisfaction from their accomplishments, and from a job well done. As leader and manager, you are also the head cheerleader. (Don't be offended, we know this isn't often spelled out exactly in your job description, but it certainly is implied in the measure of your effectiveness in most executive's minds.) You are accountable for the esprit de corps, the attitude, the feeling in your work area. (See Question 13 on organizational culture.) And a positive group spirit is achieved by the celebration of your successes. (OK, it's true that having a well-managed department, good communication skills, and a few other issues play a part as well.)

- You've got to know what success is if you are going to celebrate it. Successes are any events, changes, or behaviors that show you are moving toward your vision and acting in concert with your values. These may be incremental and small changes (all the physicians located their charts today) or more significant (we were able to discharge all the patients with DRG 207 two days earlier than expected in the month of June).

- Team successes germinate from the strengths of each member of the team (including your own). Write down what you value most about each person (this can be done with yearly evaluations, but it's even better if it's communicated verbally as well as in a birthday or holiday card such as, "I appreciate your great sense of humor when things get tough.").

- Give positive feedback (frank and honest and with sufficient detail) as often as possible. It's impossible to give too much, unless it's insincere. Part of the magic here is that when you are *looking* for the positives for giving feedback, you'll see them more clearly and help the rest of the team see them as well.

- When things go wrong, look at the bright side. (Your mother used to say "It's always darkest before the dawn" and you probably wanted to strangle her.) However, it *is* possible to draw something good from most situations, i.e., a serious error such as a patient fall and a resulting lawsuit may cause people to become more careful and thereby avoid incidents in the future. An altercation with a physician that resulted in a health care professional being humiliated may be used to teach the physician to communicate appropriately, and the health care professional to cope with conflict in a productive manner.

- Broadcast and publish your successes. Be sure the administration and the public relations department know about a spectacular recovery, a record number of treatments, an especially good safety record. Tell everyone about the improved and nearly perfect error rate or the absence of pressure sores. Let everyone know about the letters from satisfied patients or physicians.

- Use symbols to celebrate your successful work. Come up with a group slogan and logo, create fun lapel pins, T-shirts, or posters. Become obvious about your positive group identity.

- Build relationships through play. We need and deserve recreation. Whether your group likes parties, tennis or volleyball, or a potluck lunch, these are important celebrations. In health care we are often too serious. Recognize the value of humor and play in coping with daily stressors. (See Question 72.)

Clapping with the right hand only will not produce a noise.

MALAY PROVERB

REFERENCE

DePree, M. (1989). *Leadership is an art*. New York: Dell Publishing Co., Inc.

Are There Simple Strategies for Dealing with Those Difficult People?

MOST MANAGERS BEGIN their careers fascinated by the challenges of working with people. However, when some of the challenges along the way are personified in the form of difficult people, we begin considering other vocations, such as ant farming in a solitary log cabin in the mountains—anywhere—to escape!

Just as we know that the flu can spread quickly through the personnel in our organizations, the "difficult people diseases" may be even more debilitating! While flu may increase the level of absenteeism and create staffing shortages, the DPDs may cause frustration, turnover, and poor quality of care for our patients as well as headaches for managers and coworkers.

When we treat a communicable disease, we implement a step by step process: implementation of universal precautions, identification of the disease, and treatment with specific therapeutic agents. Although coping with difficult people is less clinically exact, the process is very similar. First, we obtain cultures and conduct other diagnostic tests to determine which disease we are fighting. When dealing with difficult people, recognizing the problem and labeling it as a disease is half the battle! We can then identify and laugh at the symptoms under the label, understand their origin, recognize when the shoe fits us, and begin to cope effectively with the behavior as a defined problem. (As each DPD is introduced in this chapter, we'll identify the markers of the affliction.)

Throughout the treatment process, we use universal precautions and barriers to avoid contamination with the offending organisms. As health care providers dealing with difficult staff members or coworkers, we may attempt to use distance or withdrawal as a barrier. Avoidance of most difficult people is nearly impossible and will only cause them to increase and augment their negative behavior until they feel heard. Effective universal precautions you may use to prevent the spread of these syndromes will be discussed in the following answers.

Treatment of each affliction depends on the nature of the symptoms. We don't list protocols for all the possible DPDs, but you'll be successful by following our prescriptions and using your creativity in combining treatment regimens. In all cases, it's essential to remember that most people don't *try* to become ill with biological disease, but are reacting to an invading organism. Similarly, most people don't *want* to be miserable and unpopular difficult people. They are reacting to "dis-ease" within themselves and their present or past personal environments. Although you can't repair their environments, you can take steps to encourage their dysfunctional behavior from spreading and causing symptoms in yourself and others.

> *Irate, upset people are like a fire burning out of control.*
> *They want us, by our emotional reaction, to give them*
> *"fuel." Don't give it to them. People find it very hard to*
> *argue with themselves for very long! Once they calm down,*
> *you can deal with the real issue.*
>
> Frank C. Bucaro

Q #29   When I hear that whine, I want to scream! How can I handle a whiner?

A   "It was just awful, the house supervisor couldn't find enough help, and of course the supplies weren't here, and if only you would plan ahead better and anticipate those sick calls, get more staff here, I wouldn't have been so frazzled, and there wouldn't have been those med errors they said I made. I sure wish I could spend holidays with *my* family!"

We preached that every person on your staff is valuable, and that good teamwork means you can capitalize on the strengths each individual member offers. And yes, although you'd rather strangle whiners than listen to them, they too make a valuable contribution. You may think their contribution to your job can be summed up in the number of antacids you consume. But keep in mind that coping with adversity makes you a better person. In case you aren't anxious to be canonized as a saint, recognize that whiners do make a specific (short term) contribution to your team. They give you a chance to teach them and others how to manage those with this affliction and how to take some personal accountability for resolving problematic issues. Sometimes there is a grain of truth in their concerns. If so, a manager may be able to glean a few kernels from the complaints for planning to improve quality. Let's determine how best to deal with those who greet you and your staff with that abrasive voice of powerlessness.

- Make it clear (a joking method is best) that whiners will be hung at sunrise. The urge to whine means there is a problem that each person can help solve. Each orientee must be given the word that when he or she identifies a problem, any discussion should be directed toward doing something about solving it.

- If someone begins to complain or whine, it is difficult to discern whether it's simply a whine or a real problem. Therefore, one must listen attentively.

- Take notes and direct the conversation to help the whiner find his or her true concerns. (Is the whiner just generally unhappy personally or is there an issue here?) Interrupt as necessary to keep on the track. Don't allow broad generalizations; require exact data. Be wary of "always," "never," and "they." These are the markers of the illness present in whiners. "Is it true that you *never* have enough help, or was it that you had a specific problem last weekend? Is this a real pattern or a one-time situation?" Without exact data, coping with the problem is like ordering antibiotics for a resistant organism without getting a culture.

- Remain calm (see Question 46) in the face of what seems to be criticism. Don't agree with allegations you haven't checked out, but be certain to write down and follow up on any issues that will need further research for solving the problem. People need to know they have been heard and will receive feedback.

- Ask the whiner for ideas for improvements or solutions. If the whiner continues to whine, ask for a written plan on how to rectify the problem, within a deadline, and plan a repeat meeting after you've reviewed the ideas. Let whiners know that they are powerful enough to be involved in solving an issue or making things better for themselves and others. For example: "What could the supervisor have done that would have been helpful?" "How about getting some more information about the supply issue by talking with the other charge nurses and the supply department? Could you come up with some possible solutions by next Wednesday when we meet?" "I think we are all concerned about the sick calls! You can be chair of a group to brainstorm what we can do about weekend ill calls." "I'd like you to examine each medication error and decide what *you* could have done differently to avoid this error occurring again. Include system problems but focus on what *you* could have done."

- Thank whiners for bringing matters to your attention. It's better to have them voice their concerns to you and work to fix them than for them to continually gripe and bring down the other members of the team.

- Help coworkers learn to assertively engage whiners in the group's process of improving life for themselves and their patients. Coach them in assertive responses to those who are afflicted with whining. "When you complain about things without having any ideas for fixing the problem, I feel depressed. I'd like you to work with all of us to help solve this problem and quit complaining without taking responsibility for some action." "Sally, when you start out the shift angry and upset because there isn't enough help, I feel abandoned. I'd like you to call the supervisor and find out if one of the on-call people could come in. It seems that you quit trying to solve the problem when you get so frustrated."

- Keep your sense of humor. When you hear a whine bubbling out of a reformed whiner's throat, tell them: "Oops, I thought I imagined a whine! But I know that you aren't a whiner, and since the last ones on this unit are now on Boot Hill, they are extinct here. What was the problem and how do you think you can contribute to solving it?" If joking or teasing won't work with this person, or if that's not in your comfort level or style of communication, respond with active listening.

Real nurses don't whine.

LEAH CURTIN

Q #30 How can I cure a tattletale?

A "The patient's family said she was abrupt with them, and then I heard her slam a door, and I couldn't wait to tell you about it so you could make her do a better job! She's always like this, you know."

A close relation to the whiners are the tattletales. These team members love to repair their own faded self-images with complaints about others, hoping that you as manager will somehow find *them* better and more acceptable. One wonders whether they thought their parents loved them, since this behavior is similar to that manifested by children craving additional recognition.

The energy used to tattle can be redirected toward improving communications and quality of service. Professional behavior within a supportive team forbids circuitous communication patterns: This means no backbiting, gossiping, or talking about others without ever confronting them. (For a lot of people, the backbiting, sniping behavior is very satisfying and gives them a self-righteous sense of power. For these people, this feeling must be replaced with an equally good feeling—being a part of a supportive, smoothly functioning team, feeling liked and cared about.)

- Recognize that the tattletale's motivation may be to feel more important, to get positive feedback and attention. Try to give positive attention frequently when not in a tattling session, to try to extinguish the behavior by decreasing the need for it.

- Be certain it is a clear part of your group culture to talk to the appropriate person when questionable behavior is perceived. All team members must know that any concerns must be addressed first to the person involved. Don't listen to the tattling unless this has occurred, except in the rare cases of harm to the patients or illegal or unethical behavior.

- Teach your staff to use assertive communications as a part of their professional responsibility to themselves and to others. Use examples of assertive communication when you discuss daily events and your interventions. For example: "I know the patient's family gave you some feedback. Did you get some feedback from Sue to ask her about what happened? When you tell her you heard the door slam, you might approach it like this: 'Sue, I heard the door slam. I am not sure if it was you or not.' If it was, then follow up with this: 'When you slam the door like that, I am concerned about whether it will upset the patients or their families. I'd appreciate it if you'd close the door more quietly. If you are venting your anger, there are other ways of dealing with your feelings without disturbing the unit's activities.'"

- Involve the tattletale in a plan to resolve the problem. Agree to facilitate discussion with others as necessary, depending on the level of communication skills and comfort of the staff member.

- If the tattletale behavior stubbornly continues despite all your efforts, confront the problem again in a forthright manner. "Joe, when you come to me repeatedly to intervene in what you've seen or heard, with negative information about your coworkers, I get concerned that you are uncertain about how to deal with these things yourself, or that everyone and everything is going wrong in our department. Let's come up with a plan so you can learn to give feedback to others comfortably but also get on with your own work."

> *To create an unfavorable impression, it is not necessary that certain things should be true, but that they have been said.*
>
> WILLIAM HAZLITT

Q #31 There's a person on my staff who pretends to be supportive of what I do, but then hits me broadside with comments in staff meetings. What can I do?

A It's been a confusing first few weeks in your job. But, all in all, you're feeling rather positive about your position and your contribution so far. People are still smiling and telling you how glad they are that you are here. Then, before you are prepared for it, a new DPD strikes! Yes, one of your staff is transformed. If you look carefully, you can see the *sniping snake* form emerging from the pocket of your employee's lab jacket. His or her remarks are often well-aimed strikes in the form of unfunny teasing, behind the hand comments, or digs. "Well, the *previous manager* had a photographic memory!" "We've *heard* about your performance reviews." "You of all people should know about miscommunication." "I was just kidding! Where's your sense of humor?"

Just as the snake strikes without warning, leaving the victim paralyzed, the grinning human sniper wishes to avoid retaliation by seeming funny, offhand, or innocent.

- Snipers, never able to live up to their own expectations, suffer with feelings of inferiority. They have an inflated idea of how the world *should* be and especially how perfect their manager should be. When they are able to cut down others by their attacks, they believe that they've done everyone a service by letting you know your shortcomings and retained a sense of power over their imperfect work environment. By not being forthright and open about their concerns, they feel that they have maintained personal safety and the ability to avoid responsibility. The wise manager recognizes the motivation for sniping as part of a DPD process and avoids angry retaliation.

- Quickly and quietly respond to the attack. Don't be aggressive in response, merely respond as if the comment were made in a positive and open manner. "What did you mean when you were frowning and shaking your head a minute ago?" "When you said the previous manager had a photographic memory, what did you mean? It felt like an attack on my ability to remember." "That statement sounded like you don't care for my communication style! Can you be more specific about what bothers you?"

- Ask the sniper to fully expend the venom by giving details about what is bothering them. If you are in a group, ask others to validate their perceptions. Allowing discussion, being open to feedback, may not take the sting out of the bite, but will help solve the problem behind the sniper's concerns. (Occasionally you'll find that the sniper's unrealistic expectations are at the bottom of this, or that they are just being impertinent for the feeling of being in control. Group members' wisdom will generally set the sniper straight, especially since they don't appreciate it when *they* are the subject of the sniper's attack.)

- Just as we've stated that whiners and other DPDs should not be tolerated, your handling of snipers will give the clear message that people who want to complain without personal responsibility will be called upon to be accountable for their actions, even if it's "just a joke."

> *He has occasional flashes of silence that make his conversation perfectly delightful.*
>
> REVEREND SYDNEY SMITH

Q #32 One of my staff enjoys telling people: "It's my way or the highway." What can I do about a bully?

A Everyone recognizes the symptoms of this DPD. Other staff flee in fear or quietly acquiesce to stay in this person's favor. The bullies always know what is right, are expert and informed on everything, and expect that any emphatic declaration will be honored immediately. They have successfully become unofficial leaders because so many people in your department are afraid to cross them. Often, the fear they inspire is used to manipulate the work situation to meet their needs; special scheduling, less stressful assignments. It's easy for you and your staff to "wimp out" when confronted with this DPD. Bullies value aggression, suffer fools poorly (fools being anyone who may have different ideas), and often feel justified in being hurtful to those who seem less competent or experienced. Their antennae perk up when they think they can spread the sequelae of their disease to orientees or new managers.

- *Never* run from a bully's attack. Stand your ground calmly.

- If necessary, use body language to show them you are not afraid and are willing to confront them and the issue. Stand up if they are sitting down, maintain the advantage by asking them into your office (your territory). Don't move in too closely, but maintain eye contact. Smiling in a relaxed manner (even if you have to fake the smile) sometimes helps.

- Keep cool by monitoring your self-generated internal messages. Tell yourself that you know you can handle this person. Tell yourself that you are in charge of your emotions and can affect the outcome.

- Listen carefully to what the bully is saying. Question him or her firmly and calmly, paraphrasing his or her points. Writing down important issues will help later.

- Ask what he or she would like to see happen as a result of your discussion. This allows him or her to think about a goal, thus focusing on reality.

- Listen to yourself. Don't be condescending, defensive, or argumentative. Your behavior will be a role model for teaching other employees how to deal with the bully.

- It's very easy to find yourself having to rescue the less confident in the group from the manipulations of the bully. Move out of the rescuer role and teach them that they must use the above steps to deal effectively with this DPD. The bully disease seeks out only those who are weak and unprepared. (See Questions 26 and 51 on empowerment and assertiveness.) Although there is risk involved in being assertive and standing your ground, there's more pain in being bullied repeatedly.

Courage is the price that Life exacts for granting peace.

AMELIA EARHART

Q #33 As much as I've tried to avoid it, I have hired a couple of marginal performers. How can I help them become stars instead?

A When it's the Fourth of July, you'd love to save your fireworks to light under this person's heels. You feel the urge to administer mood elevating drugs, but realize that in the bell curve of performance, there will always be some who don't hit the superior ratings. Is it reasonable to fire everyone that doesn't match your admittedly high expectations? What to do?

• Change your feelings of frustration to understanding. Take some time to find out your marginal performers' motivation for doing their jobs at all (See Question 34.) Are they working for money only, for survival? If you can't come up with fair monetary incentives within your organization, then consider the other points below. Are they depressed, burned out? Do they need to be involved in the employee assistance program? Are they bored and in need of additional stimulation to get excited about their jobs? Are they aware that you see their performance as marginal? (See Question 27 on coaching.)

• Be very clear about performance expectations. "I think you would normally be able to take an assignment of x patients, and complete their hygienic care thoroughly by 1:00." "I would expect that you could accurately fill ten refill prescriptions in this time interval." "I expect that each treatment room could be thoroughly mopped before you go to break." Be very graphic about the quality and quantity of work to be completed. Studies have shown that, frequently, performance problems are due to lack of understanding about the requirements, or staff members evaluating their performance differently than their manager does.

- While letting marginal performers know what you expect, ask them to tell you what they are planning to do to achieve their goals. "What changes have you thought of that you'll be making so that you can meet these expectations?"

- Discuss what you are going to do to support and help achieve that goal, and how you'll follow up. Ask for input about what would be helpful to the employee. Use exact dates and time intervals. "Our department educator will be talking with you each day at the beginning of the shift to determine how you've planned and organized your work and will give you some tips. I've also arranged for you to work with Juanita, so you can experience how one nurse is able to complete all of her work. I'll be giving you progress reports every two weeks, or more frequently. Let's set up our next meeting for Tuesday the 12th at 3:30."

- Also make it very clear what will happen if performance is not up to expectations by a certain date. "How long do you think you'll need to be able to complete all your medications and hygienic care by 3:30? Just two weeks or so? Good. We'll be meeting before then to update progress, but I will expect that within one month, you'll be completing your work on time nearly every day. If that doesn't happen, then we'll have to look at other options, such as reassigning you to a different job."

- Follow-through is essential. If you miss meetings or don't give feedback, you risk loss of improvement, loss of trust, and give the message that this person's substandard performance is OK after all.

- Recognize that not all of your team can be stars. Some may remain "competent . . . barely." Some may catch the enthusiasm and group spirit and will give much more energy to their jobs. Some will perform more consistently due to group pressure. "This is the way we do our work here! (and you'll have to do the same to fit in.)" Some will decide that they don't fit in, and find a job that is more comfortable for their skill and energy level. Some may slip below the competent line and will need to be urged to leave. (See Question 23 on termination.)

> *You can't teach a pig to sing. It only frustrates you and annoys the pig.*

> AUTHOR UNKNOWN, BUT OFTEN QUOTED TO US BY FRIEND AND
> FORMER BOSS, JIM STRAIN RN

Q #34 There are a few people on my staff that I can't seem to reach. They are not motivated to do anything! Sometimes I wonder why they show up for work. What can I do?

A Your choices are obvious to us. You can shoot them, fire them, or sit them down in a room with a spotlight and force them to tell you what's going on. No? Being "unmotivated" is another disease of the difficult people syndrome and can be extremely frustrating for the manager who truly wants staff members to make the most of themselves. You may indeed be tempted to put a fire under some of these folks, or to ask them to go darken someone else's unit, but these are not realistic choices. Let's look at some that are.

- Identify the behavior. We know, you said they're not motivated. But what do you mean by that? What behaviors are they displaying that give you this idea? To better understand, sit down and spend some time describing to yourself what specifically are the behaviors you are talking about. We tend to speak globally and to refer to behavior in generalities, which makes the issue too vague to resolve. Identify the specific behaviors of the unmotivated staff member (consider making a list) so that you know what it is you would like to see change. For example: attends few or no staff meetings; seldom assists anyone else on the unit even though own work is done; has never volunteered for a committee; does not attend inservices except when mandatory; does not read staff notes posted on bulletin boards; does not work extra shifts; and so on.

- Understand the behavior. Now that you've identified it, what's the cause? There are many motivational theories available, but we suggest that you take a look at your reluctant staff member in terms of Maslow's hierarchy. We know you remember this from Psych 101, but here's a brief refresher: Maslow, from Hersey and Blanchard (1988, p.32), suggests that there are several levels of needs that we all have and that we move back and forth through these levels, depending on our current situations. These levels are: physiologic, safety and security, social, ego, and self-fulfillment. How well do you know this staff member's personal situation? Can you apply Maslow's theory in the same manner that you applied it to your patients when determining if they were able to follow the care plan? Consider the staff person who rarely attends the staff meetings and never volunteers for a committee: Is this a single parent with three children, who needs to focus on safety and physiological needs first? This may be the person who becomes "motivated" to work an extra shift when you're short, but can't afford to commit to unpaid expectations right now.

Put another way, it's easier to understand the night shift's continuing complaints about a lack of decent food to eat (is the cafeteria closed?) and the unit being too cold (does the night shift wear patient gowns and bath blankets over uniforms to stay warm?). By not satisfying their basic physiologic needs, we do not foster a desire for them to move on to higher levels of functioning. Does the emergency room staff feel threatened and at risk when caring for violent patients? (This is a safety and security issue.) Do your staff members feel a sense of belonging—a team connection? (This is a social need.) Are you actively looking for opportunities to recognize people's accomplishments and give them pats on the back? (You're working on your ego level needs.) Do you provide opportunities for participation, for job enrichment, and for implementing new ideas? (These focus on self-actualization needs.)

- Meet with the unmotivated. Armed with your list of behaviors and an assessment based on what you do know about the individual's situation (both personally and on the job), seek to verify your assessment so that you can begin together to resolve the performance issue. Begin by assertively stating that you have observed specific behaviors that cause you concern. Be careful to avoid labels here! "Unmotivated" is a value-laden, judgmental term that will certainly raise defenses and quickly end any hopes of a positive meeting. (How would you like your boss to say, "Mary, let's talk about the reasons you are lacking in motivation"?)

- Form a game plan. Determine some mutual goals that you can both agree on and that fit with the employee's current situation. Perhaps your staff member is tuned in to the social level and greatly enjoys organizing the unit parties. But he or she can barely complete a chart and is nowhere to be found when data need to be collected for the monthly quality review. How about pairing this person with someone who finds charting a breeze, and have them work together for a shift or two. If you really know your people, you'll select someone who is on the ego level who will respond to the recognition and therefore be motivated to assist a fellow colleague. To ensure success, the social butterfly must agree to this strategy or come up with an idea of his or her own for improving the behavior that you have identified as troublesome.

• Be persistent. You're in the game of people development now, and results don't happen overnight. A continual, watchful eye and a supportive approach will be necessary to encourage the positive changes that you hope to see in your staff.

To keep a lamp burning we have to keep putting oil in it.

MOTHER TERESA

Q #35 How can I effectively manage the nurse who's experiencing constant personal crises?

A Almost every unit has had them. They can appear on any shift. You'll recognize them by the following statements: "Oh, I'm late because my brother-in-law needed me to post bail again!" "Well, this is the fourth marriage that's gone awry! Maybe I should try meeting men at church instead of the bar!" They are great people to be around; it keeps everyone else sane and entertained to hear of the latest crises in Cathy Crises' life. After all, she makes our own lives look pretty dull and manageable. And when we do have problems, she has already experienced something similar and can commiserate with us!

There's one (or more) problem(s) when working with a Cathy Crises. She may not be able to perform her work as well as the other folks because she's at loose ends all the time. Most people on the unit feel pretty sorry for her and are willing to pick up the slack she leaves behind. However, after a while, people get tired of doing her work as well as their own!

1. If your resident Cathy Crises is one who deals effectively with the chaos in her life and good-naturedly continues to be a productive employee as well as a lot of fun, you don't have a problem at all. Be happy your life is less like "General Hospital."

2. If Cathy does have performance problems that seem to come from her private life, clearly think about exactly which performance objectives are being missed. For example: Is her work getting done on time? Are details of her private life being shared in an inappropriate manner or place? Does the turmoil result in absenteeism or tardiness? Are her interpersonal communications with patients and coworkers smooth, or is she venting her frustrations with others?

3. When you have determined the need for improvement in an objective manner, plan a meeting with Cathy.

4. Begin the meeting by stating that, although you understand how stressful things have been for her recently, you have noted the following situation: "For the last three days, you've been coming in after report has begun. What are your thoughts about this situation?" It's important to be supportive while you gently insist that her performance must also be competent or up to standard.

5. If Cathy complains about how awful life is and how it inhibits her performance, talk about how important it is for her to find ways that she can continue to perform

competently despite these problems. Ask her how she may effectively deal with the pattern of crises in her life. Recommend a visit to the employee assistance professional or a family counselor as part of her plan. If a few days off seem necessary, help her arrange for the time needed to get her current problems in order.

6. At the end of the discussion, be certain that Cathy is able to restate the problem and what she plans to do about it. Reiterate that your support and assistance will be offered if needed. Don't offer any more support than you feel you want to. If Cathy is a very needy person, you'll have to place some parameters on the amount of time or effort you'll plan to expend.

7. Meet again with Cathy to reinforce the improvement in performance or to revisit the problem.

8. If similar problems recur, discuss the pattern of personal difficulties with Cathy and how these have affected her performance. It's now time to be more directive in referrals to your employee assistance, personnel, or counseling departments. Insist on it. This person may need help in dealing with abuse, chemical dependency, or other serious issues.

9. Oh oh! Put away that transfer slip! Resist the urge to move Cathy on to another unit or department. It's the chicken's way out. Your peers will thank you.

Things could be worse. The fact that they probably will get worse is no excuse for tossing away this golden opportunity to rejoice in our current situation. . . . There is always the off chance that adversity will improve our character. Since we are all the spiritual children of the Puritans (though mostly "fallen away"), we secretly believe that suffering is good for the soul. Constant chaos sort of keeps you on your toes.

LEAH CURTIN

REFERENCE

Hersey, P. & Blanchard, K. (1988). *Management of organizational behavior.* New York: Simon & Schuster.

SUGGESTED READING

Bernstein, A. & Rozen, S. (1989). *Dinosaur brains.* New York: Ballantine Books.

Bramson, M. (1981). *Coping with difficult people.* New York: Bantam Books, Inc.

Vestal, K. (1987). *Management concepts for the new nurse.* Philadelphia: J.B. Lippincott Co.

Chapter 7

Do Managers Need Manners?

WE ARE OFTEN surprised that this topic needs any discussion at all because it seems to imply that managers are exempt from basic courtesy. (Your salary status may be exempt, but that's about the only thing that is!) Attention to small details is essential in your position of heightened visibility. Every action you take (or don't take) can either be a magnified success or an overwhelming failure. Saying thanks, going beyond thanks, and looking at behavior at those "fun" organizational events, warrants that attention in detail, so we have devoted some space to these very issues.

> *Relationships. That's all there really is. There's your relationship with the dust that just blew in your face, or with the person who just kicked you end over end. . . . You have to come to terms, to some kind of equilibrium with those people around you, those people who care for you, your environment.*
>
> LESLIE MARMON SILKO

Q #36 I know that when my staff go out of their way to do something, I say thank you. What about when the boss does something nice? How should I thank her?

A Believe it or not, there are some things in your job that are easy to do. We'd like to encourage you to do one of the easier ones, as often as possible, because of the tremendous impact it will have. (Are you listening? Send money and a stamped, self-addressed envelope now to learn this important secret!) No, it's not a secret, and it's not Ph.D. material, either. It's the very simple phrase, *"thank you."*

Unfortunately, we take this very simple action and make it harder by worrying about proper form, or worse yet, we overlook it altogether. We have worked with more than our share of units whose staff members are contemplating mutiny, only to find out that their biggest gripe is that the manager never says "thanks." Is the phrase really that powerful? Well, how do *you* feel when someone thanks you? How do you feel when they *don't*? We rest our case.

Since we've established the importance of this simple action, a few pointers about the process are in order.

- Be aware of your excuses, those issues that get in the way of your well-intended message. We've heard them all, and then some. "I'm too busy, I meant to send a note, but now it's too late." "He already knows I appreciate the work he's doing." "It's part of his job, why should I thank him for doing what he gets paid for." "She'll think I'm trying to get on her good side." "My dog ate it." (No, that's homework, wrong list!) We get the idea. But if you're too busy, don't feel it's justified, or forget entirely, you are sending an even bigger message than you might think.

- Understand the message behind the thanks. What does that phrase really mean? We think it spells recognition and says that the action was noticed. Even though we do collect a paycheck for the job we do, that falls short of the motivational impact that a little personal recognition will give us. A simple "thank you" to everyone who attends the staff meeting will let them know that you appreciate their involvement, and is even more likely to encourage a repeat performance than making the meeting mandatory.

- Don't be stingy! Saying thanks costs nothing, is easy to do, and has tremendous motivational potential. Say it often! Not convinced? Well, Tom Peters wrote in his newspaper column (*Seattle Times*, February 8, 1993) that of the more than four hundred columns he had written, the one written on the need to say thanks generated more responses than any other single topic. It seems that people everywhere are starved for a little human recognition and appreciation.

- If the verbal message is so powerful, think what the written word can do. Very few people take the time to write a note anymore. Why not be one who does? We know of one manager who had to use every method of persuasion known to get volunteers to serve on a committee to develop a new chart form. When the job was done, she sent everyone a personal note of thanks. Several of the reluctant recruits told her they wouldn't mind doing it again, and when asked why, they told her it was because she had said "thanks."

- Don't treat your boss any differently on this one. We *all* appreciate a thank you, and your boss is not any different. Don't get hung up on any hidden meaning, or that the thank you must be in a particular format. Again, keep it simple, either written or verbal, but do it! This includes saying thanks for those events we tend to think of as perks: the company picnic, the holiday party, an educational retreat. For major events such as these, we definitely recommend a handwritten note. (Legible, of course!)

- Saying thanks is a form of positive feedback. Therefore, follow the suggestions for giving feedback: deliver the message in a timely manner, to the person involved, in a public or private setting. (See Question 27.)

- Keep the message straight. It's not fair to say thank you and then attach another request to the message. It will destroy the positive impact of the message". Thank you for cleaning the supply room. Now would you like to tackle the med room?" is *not* the best approach.

> *A powerful agent is the right word. Whenever we come upon one of those intensely right words . . . the resulting effect is physical as well as spiritual, and electrically prompt.*

> MARK TWAIN

Q #37 The Pharmacy Manager arranged for his primary vendor to speak to our unit about the third generation antibiotics that will be added to our formulary. This will really help the staff to be prepared when doctors start ordering these meds. Do I need to say more than thanks?

A Saying thanks is a great start, but we believe that there is more that can be done to continue to strengthen supporting relationships. Flowers, tickets to the ball game, free dinner, a weekend at your cabin . . . *No!* This is *not* what we meant. (Although we're sure the pharmacy manager wouldn't mind!) At the risk of reminding you once again of gender differences, women generally were brought up to "return the dish full." This may sound like a strange idea to men, and even stranger is the notion that when it comes to business relationships, men are more apt to put this phrase into practice. Confused? Hopefully, the following points will clear up what we mean.

- Review the working relationships you have with others. Do you rely on a few key individuals to assist you more often than others? What are you doing to keep these relationships strong and to ensure that the individuals will continue to be there for you ? Do you ask for favors from a select few? Do you *return the favor*?

- Be aware of fellow colleagues' needs. You're probably in the same boat as far as general needs, particularly when completing similar functions such as the budget, strategic planning, interviewing, performance evaluations, and so on. Not everyone is equally skilled in these areas, and you may find that you have some expertise to share and some insight or past experiences that will assist others to make their jobs easier. (We know, you have enough to do without worrying about everyone else. But what about when you would like someone to help you?)

- What are you willing (and able) to share? Being a team player is not restricted to just one level, but means that you will be willing to share ideas and contribute to the overall outcome of the team. If another manager asks you for assistance, are you willing to oblige?

- Don't keep score! We are not suggesting that you set up a "scratch my back and I'll scratch yours" network, but that the exchange of much appreciated favors is more likely to continue and to strengthen relationships if you are prepared to respond with more than a "thank you." Matching your strengths with others' needs and vice versa will make everyone's job a little easier.

The next time someone does you a favor, think what would be most strategically beneficial to that individual. For example, if the nurse recruiter sends the perfect person your way for that night shift position you've been wanting to fill, consider volunteering to help her staff the booth at the next community health fair. "Returning the dish" with a much needed piece of information or an offer to assist with strategies for a team conference, will make certain that no one goes empty-handed!

> *One can never pay in gratitude; one can only pay "in kind"*
> *somewhere else in life.*
>
> ANNE MORROW LINDBERGH

Q #38 We're planning a holiday party for the entire organization this year. Any advice on how to act, what to wear, who to be with?

A Any advice? What a brave question! We have enough advice on this sensitive subject to paper a few dozen bathroom walls! And, judging from the number of books that are written about management behavior on the social scene, we would guess that this is a topic that many people have struggled with. Therefore we find the need to say a word or two in warning. If you find that the following hard-learned suggestions are not enough to make you feel secure about your next event, we suggest spending an afternoon with Letitia Baldrige's (1985) *Complete Guide to Executive Manners*. This book has everything from what color of stationery to use for the invitation to what to say when no one else has anything to say!

The idea of a company-sponsored social gathering is appealing to some and creates enough fear in others that they would sooner have a root canal than join in the fun. In your position in management, it will be important to attend and support these functions, making certain that fellow staff members enjoy them as well. Here then, are a few pointers.

- Encourage participation in the planning of the occasion. Most organizations are trimming their budgets and eliminating some of the more common annual functions, so those that remain will be that much more important in terms of fostering a feeling of celebration and good will. If the holiday party or the annual picnic remain, be sure that there is a planning committee of representatives from the staff. Their involvement will help to ensure that people are planning activities that the majority will enjoy.

- Promote the idea! And encourage the committee members to do so as well! If the organization is taking the time and money to sponsor this event, the message is clear that there is a belief in the value of people getting to know each other outside of the working unit in a more relaxed setting. We all need a break occasionally, and more and more managers are recognizing the positive benefits of supporting a little play time. Your enthusiastic support can be contagious and may help to win over the most stubborn and serious employee, who feels the company is wasting money that could be better spent in the paychecks.

- What to wear depends on the purpose for the event. We always recommend a conservative approach: no short shorts or bikinis at the picnic (that applies to men too) and no revealing attire at any time. Remember, this is an extension of your business, and you will want to continue to project the same positive image that you are known for at work.

- A word about behavior. (That *is* what you asked!) There are many tales told about the company office party or the picnic where Henry got drunk and told off the boss. If alcohol is available, moderation is the key. Our best advice would be to avoid it altogether, but you may find that one drink is relaxing and adds to the *spirit* of things. (Pun intended!) Just be certain that you know your limits, and if there is any doubt, have a spouse or close associate be your gatekeeper.

  Stay in character. There is nothing more confusing and upsetting to your staff than to see a boss who gets carried away with the moment and acts out of character. If you are serious by nature and are not known to have a sense of humor, this is not the time to become the life of the party. Be yourself, naturally, and act as you feel most comfortable.

- Keep the conversation social. Often it is tempting to take this moment when you finally have the boss's ear (worse yet, the ear of your boss's boss) to start talking about the budget cuts or your latest idea for quality improvement. Save that for the office and concentrate on sharing the more fun-natured and social side of you. The same is true for your staff. An employee may see this as the perfect opportunity to discuss Martha's latest run of medication errors or the fact that Dr. Jones has made sexual come-ons to the new nursing assistant. A polite reminder that this is not the time or place and a change of the subject will get the party back on course.

- Mingle . . . mingle . . . mingle! This is a great time to get to know some of the other folks on the team. Don't get stuck in your own little group for comfort. Too often we've seen the managers all gather together like a support group at an encounter session! Venture out and talk to everyone you can! If conversation does not come easily to you, and you feel reluctant to make the first move, plan a few topics before the party. Scan the entertainment section, attend the latest movie, be up on the latest headlines, so that you have a few ideas to use when opening the conversation. Just stay away from business!

- Say thanks—to the boss, to the party planners, to the staff for coming. (And a special thank you to your spouse or partner for their support as well!) Did you have fun? You may want to have your own unit party soon!

If only we'd stop trying to be happy, we could have a pretty good time.

EDITH WHARTON

REFERENCES

Baldridge, L. (1985). *Complete guide to executive manners.* New York: Rawson Associates.

Peters, T. *Seattle Times* (Feb. 8, 1993).

Chapter 8

Is It Really Possible To Get Anything Done?

THERE ARE TIMES when we wish there were 48 hours in every day (and some times when we wish the day would end *right now*)! In this respect we are all equal: No matter what the position or role we play, we all have the same amount of time with which to work. Some of us are a little better at it than others, so we've included a few time management tips we've learned along the way. We will look at setting goals and priorities and tackle that often overlooked skill of delegation. Because you are going to more meetings than you ever thought possible, we will also suggest some strategies for making this a more productive use of your time.

One more note . . . none of these questions would be meaningful without also looking at *who* judges what we do and why we do it. Do you know?

> *To achieve, you need thought. . . . You have to know what you are doing and that's real power.*
>
> AYN RAND

Q #39 I seem to spend all my time fighting fires. Where's Smokey the Bear when you need him?

A The budget has to be cut 30 percent, you're about to begin a remodeling project, you're in charge of several systems changes, and now your secretary has quit without notice.

You're so overwhelmed with all these hot issues that you haven't had time to jump off the treadmill for a moment to take stock. There's been no time for designing the preventive measures that can decrease the number of fires you must fight. But it's when your job seems the most out of control that you must create a pocket of time to look at what you've accomplished, evaluate trends in the problem areas, and redefine your department's direction toward the future.

It *is* possible and necessary to get some time to reflect and reestablish your direction. It's not likely that someone else on the team will possess the same perspective; in most cases, others are looking toward you, the leader, for leadership from a more global viewpoint. You *owe it to your team* to put on your insulated fire gear and step back out of the fire zone, mentally and/or physically.

- Close doors, find a place physically apart, to be alone and to think. This statement is contrary to the management philosophy of open door policy, but it's necessary in order to create the space you need to do your job well. Let your group members know what you're doing: They should expect you to take time to reflect and plan, especially when you let them know you're taking time out because you care about them and your collective purpose. Consider the Native American belief about the need for silence to refocus, as expressed in the prayer at the end of this answer.

- Jot down all you've been accomplishing, even if the activities include dousing small and seemingly insignificant campfires. If you have trouble remembering, review your job description and what you have done in relation to those objectives. Look for threads or trends that show your main problem areas. For example, interdepartmental communications may have been a recurring issue, and you have created a new task force to work on the quality issues between your department and some of those with whom you interact closely. The work group's objectives may not yet be achieved, but they are in process. Give yourselves credit for what has already been done.

- As you evaluate trends in the problem areas, prioritize those challenges that require action. These may be evaluated and ranked according to those with an

  ☐ overall pervasive nature;

  ☐ those that, when solved, will have delivered the most potential benefit;

  ☐ those that are most quickly unraveled, or can be broken down into smaller, easily resolved portions;

  ☐ those that can be delegated handily and taken care of;

  ☐ and those that are recurring, complex issues that must be solved once and for all due to their potential for adverse effects.

- Decide what you are going to do to tackle each of the most pressing problems. Jot out a rough action plan, recognizing that you'll enlist the participation and help of the team in working toward solutions. Come up with some ideas to present and discuss with your staff for validation.

- Dream about what you would make of this group or service if you had a special "good fairy" that would grant all your wishes. Let that vision be a beginning for your future planning. For example, your organization could become the preferred provider for health care and preventive services throughout the health care continuum. Your housekeeping department could be the finest and most productive of any in your hospital, renowned for an exquisitely maintained environment and prompt, friendly service. Your unit could become the leader in providing cancer care education throughout the state. Feel free to dream outrageously!

- If you're not certain of the direction you'd like to go, get out your calendar and plan when you'll meet with staff members or other departments to brainstorm about more visions for your future. Ask them:

    ☐ What issues are most problematical to them?

    ☐ What would they like to see change in the future?

    ☐ If they could achieve anything, without reservation or restriction, what would this department look like in the next year, and in five years?

- Decide on days and times to again meet with yourself in a quiet space. Mark it (in ink!) on your calendar. This time should be as important to you as a meeting with the CEO of the organization. Even without access to a good fairy or Smokey the Bear, it's amazing how taking time out will free you up from the recurring problems and restore your sense of direction. (You may be able to put your fire extinguisher in storage for awhile!)

Oh Great Spirit, help me always to speak the truth quietly, to listen with an open mind when others speak, and to remember the peace that may be found in silence.

CHEROKEE PRAYER

Q #40 I feel frustrated by lack of progress. There's so much I want to accomplish. What are some realistic goals for a new manager?

A During the first year in a new management job, your primary goal is to remember your name, as you begin to discover what your job entails. In order to adapt to the increasing rate of change and stress in health care management, you and your supervisor will expect more results more quickly. However, you may still be getting to know staff members and systems and how to keep daily operations functioning smoothly. Trying to make your mark too quickly, feeling frustrated with the time it takes to make change occur, is a hallmark of the first year in management.

Let's take a look at some reasonable achievements during your "hazing" or initiation period. It's possible that you or your supervisor may hold higher than reasonable expectations for you depending on your experience and abilities. If so, negotiations may be in order. (Or you may wish to use this answer to state your case for fewer than 80 hour weeks!) In your first year, we expect you will have accomplished the following:

- Establish, with staff involvement, a clear mission and vision for your department.

- Discuss and create a clear set of performance standards (behavioral examples) based on the performance objectives in the job descriptions or other standards in your facility.

- Identify your major problem areas that need to be attacked. Base the priorities on their impact on quality of patient care, quality of work life, and the degree of drain on the budget.

- Plan a program designed to repair the above problems in the system, geared for making life easier for the workers and providing better quality, more cost-effective patient care.

- Begin to discuss with all staff members their own professional goals, progress, any need for improvement, and action plans to achieve those goals.

- If you are frustrated with progress, recognize that the relationships you are building with your team, with the physicians, and with other departments will take some time, especially if previous personnel (especially in your role!) have eroded any possible trust bond.

- Realize that progress toward your vision may take much longer than you expect. Don't let that be daunting; celebrate incremental steps toward making your department all you want it to be.

- If you take over a department with multiple serious problems, understand that you'll be able to deal only with the priorities first. Just as you wouldn't expect a dysfunctional family with many years of physical and substance abuse, poverty, and mental illness to become the Waltons or the Huxtables overnight, despite your skill as a therapist, you can't expect your department to achieve its full potential in a few months, despite your skill as a manager.

> *I mar the work of God by my impatience and discontent. . . .*
> *Patients won't wait to die, or better, to be made to live, and*
> *operations won't wait till I am less in a hurry.*
>
> FLORENCE NIGHTINGALE

Q #41 How can I possibly divide up my time to do my job?

A What does time management mean for nurse managers who are busy every second of their 12-hour work days? To many of us, time management is merely using an appointment calendar and a "to do" list. Anything further may be too restrictive; after all, we could lose our creative edge! Or perhaps you are a manager who likes the pressure and adrenaline rush of being behind, because it allows your staff to realize how busy and how important your work really is. Or maybe you're even too busy to read about how to manage your time! (We've clocked it: It will take you only 1.5 minutes to read this!)

- Keep a time log for three days to one week. (We know you're groaning, just as we did! But this is an essential step so that your eyes can be opened to the realities of how your time is being spent. Nothing can be changed without adequate assessment.) Analyze your log as you would a complex clinical problem. It will help identify problem areas: unnecessary telephone calls, unplanned "spur of the moment" visitors, unproductive time.

- Make a list of your goals and number them according to priorities. Although you'll find that there will be many necessary, urgent interruptions during your day, your long-term goals will remain. For example, you may be completing a patient education project when a family is upset and demands to talk with you immediately. Obviously, you'll re-order your priorities based on your department situation, just as you would clinically. Dealing with the family effectively will certainly support some of your long-term goals as well.

- Identify your own most problematical time wasters and develop a plan to decrease their impact. For example, if office interruptions are frequent and people come to "just visit" or gossip, close the door or tell them you'd love to go to break with them, but that you're busy right now. If telephone management is a problem, use an answering machine, voice mail, or teach your secretary how to screen your calls. If paperwork drives you crazy, develop a system by which you handle paper only once: respond and return, file, or recycle it. (Some managers build paper airplanes instead of recycling as recreational therapy!)

- Each day, plan time to work on three or four urgent and necessary tasks. Using a "to do" list with goals is helpful. Be certain that tasks reflect work toward your long-term goals in an incremental fashion.

- Break inertia on large projects or tasks you've been putting off by committing yourself to work on them for 5 or 10 minutes. Then reward yourself when you've made it through the time. When you are overwhelmed, try to divide the project into portions you can handle reasonably.

- Learn to say no to extra work that won't promote your department's goals and will be neutral politically.

- Delegate effectively. See Question 43 on managerial delegation.

- Manage your calendar by plotting all your standing meetings and appointments. Determine how best to use your discretionary time: Be certain your activities will promote goal attainment. Enter deadlines on your calendar for project steps. For example, by April 15, allocation of FTEs by shift should be done; by May 1 the rough draft of the budget should be complete.

- You are in charge of how you spend your time and your life. Although all of us are impacted by our environments and the behavior and needs of others, we must respect our goals and the time required to do our job. Too often, in an attempt to be flexible, open, and service-oriented, we tend to put our work on hold in response to others. Make each activity a reasoned choice on your part.

- *Block out time for yourself, for planning.* You're responsible for charting the course for your department; allocating the time necessary for that process is essential to your success.

- Do people really implement all of these ideas? Yes! And you'll find those people in top executive roles in highly successful businesses. As simple as our answers may seem, it takes some time to actually implement them. It does take time to save time.

There is never enough time, unless you're serving it.

MALCOLM FORBES

Q #42 People say managers are always in meetings and I certainly attend my share. How can I make the most of this time?

A It's been estimated that the average manager (and none of us are average!) will spend 10 hours per week in meetings (Mackenzie, 1990, p. 136). Over 90 percent of managers feel that half their time in meetings is wasted. Let's do a little math here: At 5 hours per week for 50 weeks (we'll give you a 2-week vacation from all those meetings!) that's 250 hours per year that you are wasting! What you could do with that time!

Think about the last meeting you attended. Whether it was the monthly parent and teacher organization at your child's school, the weekly mandatory department manager's meeting, or your own staff meeting, did you feel a sense of accomplishment when it was over? Or did you walk out of there with a sigh of relief, glad it was over till next time?

Believe it or not (we *know* you believe *us*), there are some very easy steps to take to make certain a meeting stays on course and accomplishes an objective. We haven't quite figured out how to get you out of meetings entirely, but we can help you to make them more productive. Whether you're running the meeting yourself or attending one, you can insist on the following steps. (But hey, it's only 250 hours. . . .)

- Use an agenda. It's a little difficult to track the progress of a meeting without a road map. Creating an agenda requires that there be an established purpose to the meeting and helps to reduce those meetings that are held because: "We always get together on Friday"; "We just need to touch base"; "We'd better have a meeting to see how we're doing"; and so on. It's really ideal to distribute this agenda a few days before the meeting so everyone will have a chance to prepare. (Think of it as a sales notice—maybe you'll increase attendance!) And don't forget, if you're participating, but not leading this meeting, *ask* for an agenda.

- Start on time. Sounds pretty simple, but meetings seldom start on time. Does your organizational culture allow you to straggle in to a meeting 10 or more minutes late, only to find the meeting has not started yet? Arriving late, regardless of common practice, demonstrates a lack of respect for the time of all those who are attending. And failing to start on time makes the same loud statement of disrespect on the part of the manager.

- Expect participation. The point of any meeting should be to have a meaningful, active exchange among the participants regarding an identified issue or set of problems. Let people know that you expect them to be prepared and to share in providing input regarding the matter at hand. (This is not the time for a short nap!)

- Define the purpose. If the intent of a meeting is purely informational, you may want to consider another effective means of communication. Electronic mail, short memos, or conference calls may do the trick instead of getting everyone together in one room. Clarifying the purpose will also affect attendance. Is this a mandatory meeting for very important changes in the admitting system or the weekly "We need to have a meeting every so often, and this is it" type of meeting? How many meetings are held where no one has given any thought to what the outcome of the meeting should be? Too often, we call a meeting, or attend one, without first determining what we hope to achieve. Sounds like a waste of time to us!

- Do your homework. As females, one of the hardest lessons we learned was that men typically do most of the work planned for a meeting *before* a meeting actually takes place. Phone calls are made, conversations are held in the lunch room and in hallways, and positions are established before the meeting. This is an alien practice to most females, who expect to address the issue at the meeting. After all, that's what you're having one for, right? Male or female, it doesn't hurt to do a little homework (call it politicking if it makes you feel better) to assure a more productive meeting. Know what the issue is, and how some of the other members feel about it before the meeting starts.

- Apply all of the above strategies to your own staff meetings. They are important times, yet often plagued with attendance problems and the feeling of being just nonproductive gripe sessions. Post an agenda, assign items to key staff members so that they have an active part, and above all, determine the desired outcome *before* you post the meeting.

The length of a meeting rises with the square of the number of people present.

EILEEN SHANAHAN

Q #43 Somewhere I read that management is getting things done through others. How do I do that and still feel satisfied with my job? Can I count on others when it's easier to do it myself?

A One of the hardest skills for anyone to master is that of working with other people. It may seem fundamental but, in fact, delegation is one of the areas in which most managers express having difficulty. Basically, it's tough to take the time to find someone else to do part of the job, and to do it to your exacting standards. But we would be willing to bet that you have already found out that you *cannot* do all there is to do and remain sane too. What's the solution?

- Understand your personal barriers to the process of "letting go." We mentioned a couple of the common ones above. Here are a few more to consider: the practice of nursing is being diminished as we "give away" more and more tasks (losing control); the job will not be done right (perfectionist); it's faster and easier to do it myself; I feel guilty at being unable to do it myself (supernurse). Or, perhaps it's even more personal: I feel guilty when everyone else is so busy already; no one will like me; people will think I don't know what I'm doing. Do any of these hit the mark?

- Identify the advantages. If you're going to buy this idea of investing time to delegate work to others, you'd better be able to see some of the advantages. One of the best and most satisfying advantages that we can offer comes from a statement made by Fred Pryor (1988) during one of his management presentations: "Management is getting things done through others, *while growing them in the process*." We've worked with many frustrated staff members who feel that they are not valued and trusted because the unit manager doesn't allow them to do anything new or different or, worse yet, to use the skills that they have been trained to use. Staff development can be a rewarding and long-lasting benefit to appropriate delegation.

  We're certain that you can think of other advantages as well, but to get you thinking in a positive direction, here are some of the many benefits we've been told of by excited staff members: more of a sense of "team"; more time to do what only I can do; less frustration as no one feels overburdened; and, ultimately, better patient care.

- Follow what we call **The four rights of delegation**. Just as we all know the five rights of medication administration, knowing the four steps to delegation will help you to be more successful in working with others. We will present a brief overview of the four rights; for more detail and support you may want to reference our *American Journal of Nursing* series (Hansten and Washburn, 1992) on clinical delegation.

  ☐ *The right task:* With all of the current changes in care delivery systems, it's hard to keep up with job roles and who can do what. During the nursing shortage, we were tempted to exploit certain roles and take advantage of those folks we could rely on the most. Licensed practical nurses were asked to take on additional duties that, under closer examination, were outside their scope of practice. Be sure when you are considering someone for a task that they have, or will be provided, the training to do the job, and that you do not cross any legal limits. The nurse practice act, a list of validated competencies, and your own policies and procedures will assist you here.

  You have many other duties that are not in the clinical arena and would be easily delegated to personnel who show an interest and an aptitude in the task. For instance, you might select one person from each shift to oversee the scheduling of that shift and you might have an individual review the time cards for that shift as well. Be creative in your approach! The likely candidate for these jobs is the charge nurse, if you use that type of delivery style. But why not ask the unit secretary to take on this job? Or a nursing assistant who has expressed an interest in learning new things? Or why not rotate the tasks every two months so that more people can learn and understand the importance of completing schedules and time cards?

  ☐ *The right person:* This goes hand in hand with the right task. Indeed, it's a matching game to select the right person for the right job. In some cases the choice is obvious. For example, the administration of intravenous medication belongs only to licensed personnel and would not be delegated to a nursing assistant. The person you know is motivated to become a clinical specialist may be the perfect preceptor. In all cases, you will want to select the person who is qualified in terms of training and competence to do the delegated task. There will be many gray areas here, depending on the focus of your unit and the type of patients you have. Student nurses, nurse extenders, resident nurses who have not taken the board exams yet, and patient care technicians will all have varying levels of competence. Making the right choice will be guided by your policies and the current style of practice on your unit. (Don't forget the Nurse Practice Act!)

☐ *The right communication:* A clear and concise description of the objective you have, as well as parameters for follow-up, will be essential to successful delegation. How many times have you heard these frustrated remarks: "I thought you just wanted me to watch Mr. Jones. I didn't think you wanted me to bathe him too!" "You asked me to do the time cards, but I didn't know what to *do* with them!" "Yes, I collected all the patient meal trays. You wanted me to write down the I/Os too?" The National Council of State Boards is very clear about your realm of responsibility here, and it has a terrific definition of supervision that spells out what we mean by the right communication. The definition has two parts: (1) initial direction and (2) periodic inspection of the performance of the individual. In giving the right initial direction, you are providing the communication necessary to complete the job. Ask yourself what you would need to know to complete a task to help you plan your initial direction for that task.

☐ *The right feedback:* Part two of the above definition of supervision is periodic inspection. When you are working with someone, you want to know how you're doing. The same is true when someone is working for you. Don't overlook this important final step in the process. Sometimes all that's needed is a simple thank you. Other times will require you to gather more detail as you explore the differences between what you expected and what really happened. Feedback on both sides can help to correct any mismatches that you might make and will make the process easier the next time.

Remember, you are still in control when you follow these simple steps. You have not lost the essence of your job, but enhanced it through the growing performance of others.

Tell me and I'll forget
Show me and I may remember,
Involve me, and I'll understand.

CHINESE PROVERB

Q #44 Sometimes this job seems like it's too much to handle and I *know* whatever I do is not going to be right. Any suggestions?

A You know you have an inner voice that speaks to you almost constantly. (Some of us have more than one, and then we *know* we're in trouble!) Unfortunately, for many of us, the conversation we hear most often is negative in tone and critical in nature. "Why did I make that stupid remark?" "I wish my hair looked better—I wonder if anyone noticed that bald spot, or those gray hairs?" "My skirt is getting too tight—I'll never lose those five pounds." And so it goes, as we mentally set the stage for less than positive outcomes. It takes a conscious, committed effort to "change that tape" and focus on the positive aspects of you.

Changing your self talk completely can seem like an overwhelming task. (And with your heavy schedule, it's probably the last thing on your list of priorities.) Is it worth the effort? Well, consider the very important role you play in your position. People are looking to you for leadership, you're in the spotlight, and more than ever you need to appear confident and self-assured. If there's a little voice inside saying, "You can't do this, you're an impostor, and this is too much for you . . . " then you will prove that voice right! What you need and all successful leaders have is the ability to visualize positive outcomes and tone down the negative tape "inside" your head. (We're making big assumptions here that this fits for most of you.) What we've found through experience is that while we can all easily focus on the negatives, the true leaders and coaches always keep their eyes clearly focused on the best possible outcome.

- Face each event with a clean slate. Remember the first time you tried a new skill and it didn't go smoothly? (Never? Well . . . then try to imagine giving an injection for the first time and having your hands shake so much you hit the bone . . . or maybe the first time you made a presentation to the board and you forgot what you were going to say . . .) What we tend to do with these experiences is to store them in our private little collection of top ten hits, and then replay the tape when faced with giving another injection, or another presentation, or whatever you personal favorite is. To get out of that trap, and to make certain history doesn't repeat itself, approach the event without reliving any history and move on to step two.

- Visualize the event in your mind as you would like it to happen *before it happens*. Athletes know this a tried and true coaching technique—used because it works! Runners will visualize winning the race, jumpers will see themselves clearing the bar. You can see yourself giving a presentation that is well received as you speak in a clear, confident manner. Sound too Pollyanna? Consider the alternative of being locked into a replay of your worst performance—will that inspire you and give you the confidence to achieve what you really want? We think not. We remember asking one successful department manager if the selection for a new product line was a good idea right now. His response was, "I wouldn't consider starting a new project if I *thought* it was going to fail."

- Talk to yourself in a positive manner. By now, you've probably realized that you are in a prime spot for criticism from all sides. Be your own cheerleader! Set a target of telling yourself three positive things you did today as you turn out your office light and head out the door.

- Replay your successes. Just as we know you hold your most difficult moments under the microscope, give your best performances the same scrutiny. What worked and why? Then hold that thought so you can do it again. If it didn't go exactly as you had visualized (let's face it, not all the doctors are going to give you a standing ovation), replay the scene as you would like it to have been. Hold that thought!

Man is what he believes.

ANTON CHEKOV

Q #45 Why is there never time to do it right in the first place, but always time to correct it?

A In a time when everyone from the administrator to the housekeeper is focused on cost effectiveness, time management, and the bottom line, this is an appropriate question to ask. Who defines *it* and *right* in the first place?

In management we learn that to do things right is to manage, and to do the right things is to lead. And when evaluating the job performance of your staff, you will decide if an employee is effective (doing the right job right) or simply efficient (doing the job right, but not necessarily the right job). Have we lost you yet, or are you on the "right" track?

The point of all this rhetoric is to remind you of something you already know, but need to have validated periodically to assure yourself that your focus is correct. There are, and always will be, many people standing in line to judge your performance and the performance of your staff. But in our quest to create the most effective and efficient nurses by revising job descriptions, upgrading educational requirements, and designing staffing models that would make Florence proud, we must not lose sight of the primary reason for our existence.

Many hospitals have begun to create what have been creatively titled "patient-focused" care units. This confuses us somewhat, since we thought that was what we were all doing all along. But a closer look at our organizational emphasis proves us to be wrong. Getting things done, doing things right, and being efficient have long since replaced the idea that we are solely focused on *patient* care. Times for vital signs, obtaining lab samples, bathing, meals, linen changes, and so on have been established to meet the system and organization needs and often have been counter to the patient's desires or best interests. Readjusting your focus—the focus of your team or the unit you manage—to meet the needs of your primary customer is no easy task. But there are some key points that may assist you as you continue your quest to do things right.

- Determine your anticipated outcome. We are all shifting the emphasis in our quality management programs from process to outcome. The same principle applies here: Think first about what you expect to achieve from the work you are planning. We have become so good at being task oriented, that we often focus simply on the task itself. Many of us have a mental checklist of things to do today, or on this shift, and we mentally cross them off or actually write them down for the pure satisfaction of drawing that black line through the completed item. But when we concentrate on the list, we often miss the overall picture of the *results*.

Need an example? Think about patient outcomes. We are always asking staff members to set goals with the patient that are based on assessment of his or her needs, wants, and abilities. How does this work on your unit? When elderly Mr. Smith is admitted to the floor with the diagnosis of back pain/rule out ruptured disc, he is settled in bed and an IV is started at a TKO rate, pending further orders. Do you automatically place him on I/O q 8 hrs because of the IV? What outcome would you expect from this intervention? How many staff members will be involved in measuring Mr. Smith's intake and output, recording the amounts on a worksheet and then on the chart, totalling the final measurements, and writing this on the Kardex, or entering the order in the computer or on the chalkboard under "daily I/Os"? What is the outcome that Mr. Smith can expect from all of this attention?

Sometimes we create work and use lists that serve to monopolize our time and make us feel busy. Our guess is that you are already pretty busy, but are you achieving your goals? Think of your job in terms of outcomes, in terms of the results you want to see, and move back from there to define the steps to take to achieve them.

- Be aware of organizing your work by tasks. You know the ones we mean: write a memo to the staff about the upcoming evaluations; schedule a staff meeting; complete the staffing schedule; place an ad for the night shift opening. Looking at tasks in this manner, it would be difficult to prioritize which ones are most important and need attention. Think of the outcomes you wish to produce and your list will take on more meaning. Do you want to reduce registry and overtime on your unit? (Place that ad *now*!) Is there anything else you could be doing to achieve this result as well? Have you prepared the staff for the upcoming evaluations? (So sending the memo is nice but not really essential.) We're sure you get the idea—concentrate on results!

- Determine who will benefit from the outcome. This brings us back to the beginning, to the idea that many people will sit judgment on your actions. But who will benefit? We think this is the most important focus for our efforts: the realization that we truly are here for the betterment of those entrusted to our care. It is those individuals who will determine whether we are doing the right things right.

Decide what you want, decide what you are willing to exchange for it. Establish your priorities and go to work.

H. L. HUNT

REFERENCES

Hansten, R. & Washburn, M. (1992). Time and organizational management. Workshop developed for the Center for the Advancement of Healthcare and Educational Services, University of Phoenix.

Hansten, R. & Washburn, M. (1992, March–August). Working with people [column]. *American Journal of Nursing*.

Mackenzie, A. (1990). *The time trap*. Delran, NJ: Newbridge Book Clubs.

Pryor, F. (1988). *How to turn your work group into a winning team*. Workshop by Pryor Resources, Inc.

Chapter 9

How Can Communication Account for So Many Problems?

IT'S BECOME A pat phrase, like a mantra, that we hear applied to almost every tough situation: "We're having a problem with communication." Variations include the ever popular: "It's not our fault communication got screwed up." No matter what, we can trace the root of *any* problem back to that pesky issue of communication. Verbal or nonverbal, written or taped, communication is the key to all of our problems. So, it is only understandable that you would have some questions regarding this topic; we have included some of the more strategic answers here.

A word of warning: We will be covering your questions on criticism, gossip, persuasion, memo writing, and assertiveness. This is not meant to replace the theory and format that is the foundation of basic business communication. If you find you are having difficulties in this area, we suggest perusing a copy of *Business Communication: Strategies and Skills* by Richard C. Huseman, James M. Lahiff, and John M. Penrose, Jr. (1991) or checking at your local bookstore or library for the latest book on business communication.

If you have anything to tell me of importance, for God's sake begin at the end.

SARAH JEANETTE DUNCAN

137

Q #46 As a manager, how do I handle criticism? I seem to be getting it from all sides, and I thought I was the one who was supposed to be the manager?

A Criticism, an emotionally charged term, is certain to push the defense button in all of us. As our kids often plead, "Don't criticize us!" And they would be the first to agree that everyone doesn't love a critic. Theodore Roosevelt made the denouncement a little more eloquently, "It is not the critic who counts; nor the man who points out how the strong man has stumbled, or where the doer of deeds could have done them better. The credit belongs to the man who is actually in the arena. . . ."

Where is the credit for today's managers in the health care arena? There is apparently enough criticism to go around: Physicians criticize the staff when orders are not carried out; the staff criticizes management when staffing is tight and the raises are less than desired; and the boss criticizes you for not running a more efficient unit. It seems everyone is a critic! But who needs it?

No matter what position you hold, or the role that you play (and that includes the highest executive), an honest appraisal of your behavior or performance is important for you to continue to develop and grow in your abilities. Sounds a little like a parent telling you that vegetables are good for you (and you didn't buy that line either). Criticism, like broccoli (now, that's stretching it), is a negative dish, and is frequently equated with harsh or severe judgment. Usually delivered in a charged personal encounter, this is not the feedback required for positive growth! How do you handle this, and manage at the same time?

- Isolate the issue from the anger. If you are the target of a critical comment like one of the examples above, this will be your most strategic and difficult task. As the physician carries on about the lab work that is not done, it's important to recognize that the real message here is *not* that you are inefficient, but that a process that was ordered was not completed. Depersonalizing the situation by keeping your sense of self separate from the exchange will allow you to focus on the very important and correctable situation. As a manager, however, you will be *deservedly criticized* for *not* taking steps to follow up and investigate the cause of the physician complaint.

- Watch the defense. All too often, we have seen people respond to criticism with defensive comments. "It's not my patient." "The night shift left too much to do." "We're too busy to be able to do everything!" It's natural, when under attack, to want to defend and get yourself off the hook as quickly as possible. Unfortunately, this only tends to accelerate the critic and to avoid discussion of the real issue, as you squirm in discomfort, feeling embarrassed and ineffective. It's not a pretty sight, and one of our least pleasant memories!

- Acknowledge the comment or criticism, state that you will look into it if appropriate, and follow up as necessary. Criticism does not require excuses but is a call to action or a very useful red flag to alert you to a problem that needs your attention. (Although sometimes we feel that there are too many flag wavers out there and we'd like to . . . oops, are we taking this too personally?)

- Invite critical appraisal of your performance as a manager. One of the most effective strategies we know is to beat the other guy to the punch, so to speak, by asking for a little honest feedback about how things are going. Many of your staff members, as well as your peers, and certainly upper management are observing your actions and making their own personal evaluations anyway. Keep them honest by asking them to share their observations with you. This takes a secure and confident individual (which is why you are reading this book), but the benefits are tremendous. The person you've asked feels valued in a new way, and you gain some insight from another perspective regarding what you are doing. A word of caution here: Don't overuse this strategy and start asking everyone how you are doing—word will get out that you are either insecure or looking for praise!

- To answer the second part of your question, yes, as a manager *you* are also supposed to be the one giving critical appraisals of those employees who report to you. This issue is covered in greater detail under performance evaluations, but there are a few key points worth mentioning here. Make sure that your criticism is valid and your intention honest. Righteous indignation has its place but will seldom bring the desired results you hope to achieve. Evaluate the price of that fleeting moment of power when you communicate in anger versus the potential outcome of a more calmly delivered appraisal. Can you afford the short term satisfaction of sending a pie into someone's face?

- Remember, criticism flows more easily downhill. Studies have shown that the higher you go in the administrative tree, the more constricted the feedback channels become. The risk of reprisal becomes greater with every step up the ladder, isolating you from the important feedback that you need and creating a great reluctance to share observations with colleagues and superiors. Consider your past experiences. Were you comfortable telling the physician that his angry outbursts were alienating the staff and hindering effective patient care management? Have you told your supervisor that his lack of consistent communication with the employees feels like a lack of support? These are tough topics, we know, but we know you can handle them with a calm, direct approach!

Criticism is like champagne: Nothing more execrable if bad, nothing more excellent if good.

CHARLES CALEB COLTON

Q #47 Criticism is one thing, but how about all these negatives?

A You have probably heard the old saying, "If you can't say anything nice, don't say anything at all." (We're sure that was your mother talking, or maybe you have taken the opportunity to invoke this wisdom on someone you know.) Just as likely, you have been the target of comments that were not so nice, and that's why you've asked this question. (Didn't these people have good mothers?) Opportunities for complaints and criticism are unfortunately abundant in today's negative society. How well you handle the verbal slings and arrows can play a large part in your professional well being.

Fortunately, this is a topic that has been studied at length. There are hundreds of books written on how to deal with difficult people, manage conflict, and deal with the downers in life. Through research and the school of experience, we've developed the following steps to help in dealing with the less positive comments that may come your way.

• Establish a positive environment. Hallway confrontations and loud arguments in public work areas are disruptive to all. The environment becomes clouded with bad feelings and the negative atmosphere is contagious. When approached by someone who is obviously upset or angry, a good move is to acknowledge your willingness to listen while guiding him to a more suitable, private place. (The end of the pier is our first choice, but that would mean you weren't open to what might be a legitimate concern.) If you are trapped in a committee meeting when someone decides to take aim at your new proposal for weekend staffing in the oncology unit, acknowledge the comment and offer to discuss this after the meeting. If feedback about staffing is the focus of the meeting, then proceed to the following steps.

- Listen empathically. Whether a complaint, criticism, or insult, it is important to understand

  ☐ that the person feels strongly about the issue;

  ☐ what the issue is; and

  ☐ why the feeling is there

  Would you feel the same way if the situation were reversed? (Of course you would, if your mother was a patient in the hospital and she had waited for a pain shot for hours.)

- Pause and reflect. This is no doubt the most difficult step to achieve. Natural instinct will tell you to defend yourself or the situation or, worse yet, to respond in anger. You feel attacked, and the biological surge of adrenaline is preparing you for "fight or flight." Now, more than ever, taking a few moments before you respond will allow you to frame the best response. The point should not be to take your best shot or to impress anyone with a clever retort. But speak when you are angry, and you'll make the best speech you'll ever regret.

- Depersonalize the issue. Easier said than done when you've just been made the target of a patient's complaints that his call light went unanswered for twenty minutes and he could hear nurses laughing at the desk. As he continues his tirade, wanting to know who the boss is around here because this is certainly no way to run a hospital unit, you feel your anger rising. Keeping your cool now and looking at the real issue provides opportunity for resolution, while an instant defense may bring short-lived gratification and escalate the issue. We know you'd really like to tell the patient how difficult running a unit is these days, and perhaps he'd like to take over so that he could control the nurses a little better and improve the service around here on a limited budget! Oops—better go back to the previous step!

• Present your response frankly and assertively. It is seldom necessary to return a negative attack. Such action will only serve to move you into an argument, best described as an opportunity to miss the most important part of the conversation. Again, remember to focus on the issue, not the person (you or Mr. Negative). A calm, clear statement of your perception of the problem will go a long way in dealing with a negative comment.

> *Before you give somebody a piece of your mind, make sure you can get by with what you have left.*
>
> ANONYMOUS

Q #48 It's not unusual for the team to sit around and gossip about someone. This makes me feel uncomfortable, and I'm not sure how to handle it. Any suggestions?

A We're not surprised that you feel uncomfortable. The potential for harm becomes more apparent the farther up in management you go. More than one career has come to a premature end by the instigation of a harmful story that may not even have been true. So, grab some cookies and pull up a chair as we elaborate on your mom's well worn advice, "It's not nice to talk about other people."

• Understand the reason for gossip. Someone is seeking attention, and it is usually the person who feels that the sensational and personal message they are dying to share will put them in the limelight they crave. Unfortunately, this visibility is gained at the expense of someone else. Protesting the target and correcting the attention seeker come under the heading of your additional duties if this involves a member of your staff or a colleague.

- Resist the temptation to add your information, even if you know it is true. In a management role, you are a highly visible role model. Take advantage of this opportunity to demonstrate your true leadership qualities by doing what Mom taught you—defend the target by stating,"I don't think you're being quite fair," or "I don't think that's something we need to discuss." This will tell your staff clearly that gossip is not an acceptable pastime.

- Remember, "If they talk about someone else, they'll talk about you too." Sage advice from dear old Mom that proved all too true. If your staff members see you engaging in the discussion of personal issues and rumors, they will easily draw the conclusion that you will talk about them in this manner as well. Is that the message you want them to have?

- Encourage the members of your staff to "send the mail to the right address." (Sharon Cox's (1989) workshop advice.) Too often, a group of staff members will have a spare moment and will spend it by sharing their feelings about someone's recent behavior. The story takes wing and is soon embellished by additional tales of a personal nature. Everyone loves juicy gossip, and the willing participants take off with little regard for the target. As Sharon observes, we tend to tell *everyone* else our views surrounding someone's offensive or disappointing behavior, *but the source*. Telling the person directly stops the rumor mill and just might lead to a productive correction of the problem in the first place.

- Defuse gossip by having other alternative topics ready for conversation. No matter how busy you keep the staff, there will always be time for gossip. (It's amazing how a story can get started while preparing an intravenous solution.) Be ready to suggest discussion of the latest movie, a book you have read, the new issue of "Nursing Jocularity," or even the upcoming staff meeting. The idea is to turn off the rumor mill every chance you get, with a clear and consistent message that this type of recreational conversation is not acceptable sport on your unit. Right, Mom?

> *Count not him among your friends who will retail your privacies to the world.*
>
> PUBLILIUS SYRUS

Q #49 As a staff nurse, I never had to write anything other than my charting. Now I have to write memos, reports, and everything. Is there a special way to write a memo? And even more confusing, who gets a copy?

A And you thought charting was a pain! Those of you who secretly aspire to be Hemingway will enjoy this aspect of your job, and the rest of you will sigh with dismay as you realize how much paperwork there can really be in a management position. Our biggest dream is to become like the deck on the starship Enterprise—there's *no paper anywhere!* But without Captain Kirk to guide us, we must still struggle with the need to communicate in writing. We propose some of the following suggestions to make the job a little easier and head you in the direction of a "Star Trek" adventure.

• Keep it short. (We heard that sigh of relief!) A memo should be direct, action-oriented, and brief—we are all busy people who do not have a great deal of time to spend in leisurely reading. A good rule of thumb to use here is the one page limit: If you can't say it on one page, you haven't thought through the issue clearly and are in danger of losing your reader. We know of some managers and administrators who warn their staff that if it's more than a page, they won't read it!

- Consider your purpose. Is the point you need to make clear and straightforward, such as the need to announce an inservice scheduled for Friday, or a staff meeting, or a change in policy? Some topics will require a more lengthy discussion, such as the proposal to add a visiting lounge to your unit. This should not be a memo, but a formal report that follows a different format. You may alert your boss to the need for a proposal by way of a memo, but making your case will require a much more formal final document. (And when you are faced with writing a report of this nature, be sure to include a brief executive summary on the first page that will highlight all of your main points. This *Reader's Digest* version will certainly be read—it may be the only thing that is —and you will at least have shared your view.)

- Answer the questions who, what, when, where, and why. Using this reporter's method of sharing information will keep you focused and your message complete. Don't leave the reader frustrated by announcing a meeting next Monday for a new committee but neglecting to explain the purpose of the committee (or the purpose of the meeting for that matter).

- A word about format: If you work in a large facility, you probably have an accepted style, or a computerized heading for a memo. Generally, the heading will indicate that this is a memo and may follow with:

    To:
    From:
    Date:
    Re:

to give the immediate details of the memo. Follow this heading with the body of your memo in a clear and direct style. This is not the time to be chatty or ramble on (save that for the electronic mail) but to precisely state the purpose of this piece of paper.

• A memo can be forever. One of the primary reasons for writing a memo is that it leaves a record. Just as you document patient care, the memo documents the information shared, the compliment given, the complaint issued, the warning notice, and so on. While many of these exchanges can and do take place verbally, there are times when a more permanent record needs to be established. However, a poorly written or an ill-conceived memo can have the same life span as the one that is clearly written and well-intended. Think before you write! You are contributing to your image with every word you put on paper.

   You may feel that far too many memos are written. As your desk becomes buried by a snowfall of interdepartmental memos, you may question your career choice. Surely charting was not this bad! It will take time, experience, and a liberal understanding of your organization to become comfortable with the use of memos as a means of communication.

• What about copies, carbon copies, and "blind copies"? Now that you've written your version of *Gone with the Wind,* who gets a copy? (Notice that we didn't ask who *wants* a copy!) It is only courteous to send a copy to anyone who is mentioned specifically in the memo. If you are suggesting to your boss that you and the pharmacy manager believe a new medication system should be reviewed, a copy to the pharmacy manager would be expected and would be indicated at the bottom of the memo with: c: J. Smith. ("cc" is passé now that we have photocopiers and no longer use carbon paper and carbon copies.)

Blind copies are those copies of a memo that are distributed to interested parties whose names are not listed at the bottom of the memo. This is a political tactic by which you are sharing information with someone without letting the announced receiver of the memo know. This is extremely inappropriate if you are sending a blind copy to the receiver's boss to let him or her know your position on an issue without letting the receiver know. (In fact, we think blind copies seem underhanded no matter what your reason.)

Supervisors and bosses can present their own set of sticky issues when it comes to memo copies. For instance, if your boss's boss asks you to look into a complaint and report back to him or her, which boss gets the memo? Depending on the practice in your organization, it is usually acceptable to write the memo directly to the person requesting the information, no matter what his or her position. Just be certain to "copy" your immediate supervisor. It would *never* be advisable to write a memo to your boss's superior without being asked and without keeping your boss advised. Going over the boss's head is almost always a fatal move. (So many rules—Scotty, beam us up!)

Make it so.

> CAPT. JEAN LUC PICARD, "STAR TREK, THE NEXT
> GENERATION"

Q #50 I have a great idea for changing the way the unit is organized. Any suggestions for implementing my plan?

A Yes, Yes, Yes! We love the idea of changes and improvements and the new energy that comes from the innovative approach. But we have seen many an idea stonewalled by resistance, leaving its would-be facilitator paralyzed and defeated. Before you toss your idea against this wall, review the following hard learned suggestions:

- Try your idea out on your mentor or closest ally. This person will no doubt give you confidence, support, and praise, and energize you for moving on to step two.

- Try your idea out on your strongest adversary. *What? Are we crazy?* This takes courage, we know, as you risk a great deal in sharing your vision with someone you know will not support it. What he or she will do, however, is be the best devil's advocate you could find. (An interesting byproduct might also be that he or she will be flattered that you valued his or her opinion enough to ask.) Take note of all objections. This is your worst case scenario. Can your idea survive? Do you have answers to overcome the arguments this adversary will raise? If not, it's back to the drawing board before leaping into this ice water bath again!

- Select three or four informal leaders among your staff (from all shifts please). Share your idea and ask for their suggestions. Take note of these and adapt them where you can so that this becomes *their* idea as well. Describe your timeline for moving forward and enlist their support, asking for positive and vocal participation when you take the idea to the rest of the staff.

- Determine who will be affected by your proposed change. If you want to improve a system that directly involves your nursing personnel, go one step further and analyze who will indirectly feel the impact. For example, a proposed change in documenting the vital signs at the bedside may on the surface be a great way to improve the system. But the indirect impact to the physicians who are used to a clipboard recording at the chart rack may build a Great Wall of China's worth of resistance to your proposal. Realizing this before you move ahead will allow you to include those indirectly involved in your network of allies. Repeat the same process with them, selling your idea, inviting critical appraisal, and enlisting a few disciples to support you when you translate your idea into action.

- Remember, change is slow. Be patient with yourself and your group. Carefully build a group of supporters that you can trust so that when you are ready for action, you already have a well-placed team to help you over the wall.

Good judgment comes from experience, and experience comes from bad judgment.

BARRY LEPATNER

Q #51 Sometimes people tell me I'm being belligerent when I think I'm just being assertive. How can I find the middle ground between being a wimp and being aggressive?

A The 1980s seemed to be the decade of assertiveness. People began to learn that how they communicate—the words, the body language, the setting—affects how their message is received by others. And ultimately, the quality of your communication determines the quality of your life. (Think about this statement for a minute: Isn't it true that how well you are able to transmit your thoughts, ideas, concerns, and feelings translates to a measure of success in all areas of your life?)

So let's define assertive behavior, the midpoint of the spectrum from aggressiveness to passivity. We all display various kinds of behaviors from time to time. But we'd achieve our goals and feel better about ourselves if we would use assertiveness more frequently. Assertiveness is not a weapon, and doesn't equate with stubborn, impolite, or obnoxious behavior. Sometimes, assertive behavior seems aggressive or harsh to people who are not used to openly stating how they feel in a positive manner. Those people may tend to adopt nonassertive patterns. They let others walk all over them ("Don't worry, I'll be glad to take two more patients than everyone else!"), allowing the needs, wants, and goals of others to be more important than their own. They may also play the role of the victim while gritting their teeth.

Aggressive behavior can be active bullying (such as the nurse who throws the chart and verbally degrades another department) or passive, which may be less direct and obvious. Passive-aggressive behavior would be exemplified by the 3:00 A.M. telephone call to a physician you don't like, sweetly asking for a "prn milk of magnesia order"! In either case, the aggressive person is acting with disrespect for the rights and feelings of others, acting as if he or she feels superior.

Here's a quick quiz: Label each statement below as assertive, aggressive, or nonassertive behavior.

☐ (Delivered loudly, pointing your finger at a coworker): "You are disgusting! Don't you ever pick up after yourself? You always think the rest of us are your slaves! You leave the medroom like a pigpen!"

☐ (To yourself, silently): "Oh, dear, this medroom is a mess again. I guess I'll have to clean up after Sue again. It sure makes me mad but I don't want to lose her friendship by saying anything to her."

☐ (Said in a calm voice, directly to Sue): "Sue, when I walked into the medroom a moment ago and saw all these syringes, empty vials, and wrappers I wondered what was going on?" (Await a response from Sue that confirms she's not in the middle of an emergency.) "I feel frustrated in getting my own work done when I have to pick this up before I can get started. I'd like you to throw this stuff away before you leave. Great!"

You were right if you labeled the first statement as aggressive, the second nonassertive, and the last assertive.

1. Assertiveness begins with a feeling of respect for yourself and others. You believe that you are a worthy person and have a right to express your wants, needs, and goals as equal to those of other people.

2. Take a look at your body language and how you express yourself. Listen to your tone of voice on a tape recorder; look at yourself in the mirror; ask a friend how you come across. Try to converse in a relaxed manner, with good posture (yes, it does make you look more confident!) and level eye contact.

3. Realize that you are in control of your own method of communication, but that you can't control other people's choices. You can choose to react to others and escalate your differences, making honest discussion even more difficult. Or you can accept others' styles of interaction as a product of their own backgrounds and differences and choose to interact with them in a respectful and honest manner.

4. Use "I" statements. Describe accurately your own feelings and thoughts instead of using "you" statements that will seem judgmental and put the other person on the defensive. For example: "I felt afraid when you didn't come to help with that emergency right away," instead of, "You ditched out when I needed you!"

5. Focus on factual descriptions of what has just happened: what you have seen, heard, read, or experienced. For example, "When I heard you slam that door, stating 'I'm never coming back here!', I felt angry and embarassed,"

instead of, "You're always slamming the doors and saying you'll quit! Why don't you!"

6. Tell people directly what you want them to say or do differently. Be clear; use please and thank you. For example:
"Please tell me what the problem is so we can discuss it,
without drawing attention to your anger in front of the
patients," instead of, "Can you try not to do that again?"

7. It's OK to say no! It's not necessary to come up with five
or six reasons why not. ("My cat is sick, I'm too busy, my
mother-in-law is visiting, and I really don't like you, so I
can't be on that committee.") Just be polite. "No, I am
choosing not to be a member of that committee." Feel free
to offer other alternatives. "I can offer the names of two
of my staff members who may wish to participate,
though."

8. If you are feeling uncomfortable about a decision or situation, it is assertive to say "You know, I have mixed feelings about that. I'll have to think about it before I can
make a decision."

9. As a memory jog, the assertive language formula includes:

   ☐ When you . . . (describe objectively what you have
   seen, heard, read)

   ☐ I feel/think . . . (describe how you feel or how you
   think this will affect you, others, or the health care organization)

   ☐ I want/would like . . . (describe what you'd like to see
   happen instead in objective, detailed terms)

10. Remember, if there is a problem with the behavior of another person, don't try to solve it for them. Ask them
what they think they could do to solve it.

11. Practice, practice, practice! When you practice assertive language and state, "When you . . . I feel . . . I want . . .," we feel elated and hopeful about your personal and professional success, and want you to make it a habit!

And the trouble is, if you don't risk anything, you risk even more.

ERICA JONG

REFERENCES

Bits and Pieces. Vol. No. 1, Fairfield, NJ: The Economic Press, Inc.

Cox, S. (1989). *Taking the mama out of management*. Workshop presented to the American Organization of Nurse Executives convention, Chicago, Illinois.

Huseman, R.C., Lahiff, J.M., & Penrose, J.M. Jr. (1991). *Business communication: Strategies and skills*. Chicago: Dryden Press.

SUGGESTED READING

Fruehling, R.T. & Oldham, N.B. (1988). *Write to the point*. New York: McGraw-Hill Book Co.

Chapter 10

Any New Ideas for Coping with "Unanticipated Adventures in Management"?

MAKING DECISIONS, SOLVING problems, negotiating for a win-win solution to a conflict—can't you just visualize "Super Manager" sitting at his or her desk, picking up the phone, and implementing all of the above skills with the smooth panache of a master? Although we perform all of these skills daily in our lives outside of work (yes, there is a life outside of your workplace), we don't often reflect on the processes involved when we hit a glitch in applying them.

Next time you face "unanticipated adventures in management," we challenge you to open this book and match your thought processes with our answers.

> *Life is either a daring adventure or nothing. To keep our faces toward change and behave like free spirits in the presence of fate is strength undefeatable.*

> HELEN KELLER

Q #52 What about the complex problems I have to solve? How do I make the right decision?

A In your formal education, you probably learned a zillion different methods for individual and group decision making. We have attempted to distill these models into a relatively simple framework, designed to be used as a crutch or reference when your first attempts have gone awry. *Note:*

These steps involve logic. The nuances of judgment, based on your experience, hunches, feelings, and intuition are not mentioned. Intuition has been found to be a scientifically valid tool for guiding your decision making, especially where there exists a high level of uncertainty, you are under time pressure, and there are good arguments either way. Use your intuition, but mix it liberally with the following steps!

At risk of redundancy, we hope you aren't attempting to solve complex problems alone. The active participation of staff members in solving problems that affect them not only ensures that more brain power will be expended, but improves the potential for the best results. If you are facing a lonely management problem that is personal or involves personnel issues and can't be shared with staff, consult with a peer or a supervisor for input.

- Describe the objective signs or symptoms that cause you to think a problem exists; then decide what should be happening instead. Think about what's *good* about this problem. (This allows you to think in a positive manner and frees you from being doomed to the uncreative mindset of "woe is me, life just keeps getting worse!")

- If you were able to choose the best of all possible worlds, what would be happening? Allow yourself to go beyond the restrictions you know to be in place in real life and think freely. It's fun and allows people to move beyond self-imposed boundaries such as, "We'll *never* get more money for a crazy idea like *that*!"

- Decide whether the symptoms describe a possible problem. If there is a real problem, should you do anything about it? To help you decide, ask:

  ☐ Does this problem affect me, my department, or those we serve? (If not, why are you spending your time on this? If it is someone else's problem, "turf" it to the appropriate person.)

☐ What would happen if I don't do anything? (What people will be affected if you don't, and how would this sit politically in your organization?)

☐ What will happen if I *do* try to solve it? Who is affected? (Keep in mind that if *you* are affected by this problem, and *you* care enough to expend the time to fix it, that should be enough.)

☐ Do the differences between my goal and what's really happening constitute a problem, or can I live with the shortfall?

☐ Is this problem something I *can* do something about myself or within my department?

- Name or define the problem. What isn't exactly the way you want it yet? What objective criteria will help determine if it is solved? Be as measurable as possible. For example, if the problem is solved we could see a 25 percent reduction in overtime, or fewer than two complaints per month, or a reduction in required patient care hours by 5 percent.

- Brainstorm for all the possible alternatives. (This is where it's most helpful to have those additional minds working with you on the solution.)

- Evaluate the pros and cons of each alternative solution.

- Decide which alternative has the highest cost to benefit ratio. Keep in mind the resources that will need to be expended for implementing the action steps, such as educational costs. Think about what *you* are prepared to *give* or *change* to make things improve. Think about what you are willing to *part with* or *do differently*. Important: Ask staff who are affected what *they* are willing to change to make things better. This is a well-proven method of encouraging staff to see their own accountability for solving the problem.

- Plan the steps of implementing the solution. How can you find a way to *enjoy the process* while you are doing what is necessary? (A. Robbins, 1992) Remember: Life is *now*. A scowling group who implements solutions with jaws clenched have lost sight of why they are in the profession and will diminish hope of successful resolution. Enjoying the process may mean something as simple as envisioning the surprised look on Dr. Mark's face when the labs are on the charts on time!

- Evaluate the results of the solution, using your objective criteria. At this point, if the solution isn't yet having the desired impact, check to see whether all the necessary communication and education has been done properly and thoroughly. Another law of management: These things usually take more time than you think they will.

- Revise your solutions based on your evidence. Go back to brainstorming and repeat the steps that follow. Remember: Repeated problem solving and continuous quality improvement are part of the manager's role, whether you are coaching your staff or assuming much of the responsibility for the process yourself. If everything were always perfect, why would they need to pay you?

- If you continue to experience the problem, check:

  ☐ Have I correctly defined the *real* problem?

  ☐ Are the symptoms being caused by something else?

  ☐ Did I take time to adequately research the facts?

  ☐ Have I given the problem's solutions enough time to work?

  ☐ Have I communicated well enough to all those involved?

- If there is a decision that you have to make alone, don't be afraid to make it! Indecision does not inspire your team members to follow you. They aren't sure if you know where you're going, and they won't sign up for your tour!

> *When the decision is up before you—and on my desk I have a motto which says "The buck stops here"—the decision has to be made.*

> HARRY S TRUMAN

Q #53 There's always a certain amount of conflict somewhere in our organization. How can I handle conflict creatively?

A Conflict! Merely thinking about our most recent conflicts may cause brave, heroic managers like us to shrink and feel like running away. Despite the nauseous feeling in the pit of our stomach when we envision conflict, we must recognize its value in our lives and workplace. Without conflict, problems would not be identified and solved and new creative ideas would not be perfected. Disagreement among committed professionals is as inevitable and essential as drawing a breath. In fact, the only time that we do not experience conflict is when we no longer breathe!

- Identify your most common style of dealing with conflict. In addition to the many self-tests that are available to identify conflict coping methods, you may want to reflect on the modeling of conflict resolution you were exposed to in your formative years. If the "hold it all in and blow" or "run away and hide" approaches were used in your family, you may have tendencies to adopt those methods in your own life and as a manager.

- Learn to recognize a conflict so that you can apply these principles. *Naming a situation as a conflict* in our brains enables us to work with our skills, and helps us to direct the emotional energies we may be feeling because of the circumstances. Then give the issue your full attention immediately.

- Learn to keep cool so that your brain is still engaged in re-solving the conflict. Experiment with some of the strategies we've accumulated from years of asking people how they keep a cool head. Adapt and use what works for you.

  □ Separate the person from the problem: Clearly identify the real issues and avoid thinking about the negative feel-ings you may be having about the person.

  □ Use visual images to decrease your anxiety. Envision yourself in a safe place or on vacation. To make the person less frightening, envision him with a clown hat or nose, or in his pajamas. (Some people have said they envision people naked!)

  □ Use your own self-talk to keep calm. "In a hundred years, no one will remember this day or this situation. I can eas-ily cope with these issues and this conflict. I will be suc-cessful."

  □ Take deep breaths, or take some time out. "I'll get right back to you on this."

  □ Some people still use the time-honored, Mom-endorsed strategy of counting to 10, or perhaps 100!

- Empathize with the other parties, focusing on the feeling tone. This will take some of the wind out of their sails, when they feel their emotions have been heard. "I can see that you are angry. I can understand why you would be upset." This also helps establish trust that you will respect their ideas and emotions.

- Obtain and give information assertively. Get the facts about what happened, carefully jotting down ideas. Writing down the facts will help keep everyone cool and will again show others that you are anxious to resolve the issue. Keep fact and opinion separate. (See Question 51 for assertive language.)

- Establish your mutual goals and what the other party wishes to accomplish by this conversation. Whatever you decide, reiterate your mutual goal ("We are both committed to quality patient care" or "improving staff satisfaction.")

- Ask for the other party's assistance in resolving the conflict issue. "How do *you* think we can resolve this conflict so that both of us feel comfortable with the end result?" If this step is ignored, you'll end up with responsibility for fixing things when the issue is definitely not one-sided. Some people are more than glad to create conflict but don't wish to be involved in the resolution. Encourage creativity!

- Summarize what you've agreed upon as alternatives to resolving the conflict. This is a great checkpoint to see that both parties have been involved: Do each of you have a job to do in the future? "From now on, I'll check the schedule before I try to use this room for a meeting. And in the future, you'll change your meeting to Tuesdays instead?"

- If your conflict resolution attempts have not been successful, remember that it's necessary to work with a willing participant to develop creative alternatives, and that's not always possible. Just remember, it's better to work through a few conflicts successfully and/or unsuccessfully than the alternative: no conflict, no breath!

> *Conflict is the seed of creativity,*
> *Communication the soil,*
> *Honesty and respect the fertilizer.*
>
> NORTH DAKOTA FARMER

Q #54 There have to be better ways of bargaining for what I want within our organization! How can I become a better negotiator?

A Negotiation is a necessary skill for those who wish to enjoy a long career in health care management. Negotiation goes beyond conflict resolution. It requires a deeper understanding of your own and the other party's interests, being more savvy in your ability to think critically and implement strategy. Fisher, Ury, and Patton (1991, p. xi) define negotiation as "back and forth communication designed to reach an agreement when you and the other side have some interests that are shared and others that are opposed."

What is your attitude when discussing negotiation? Those of you who work in union environments may think of union negotiations. Although we are not specifically targeting union bargaining in our answer, the principles apply. Many managers refrain from negotiating because they feel afraid of failure, of losing, or because it seems to be a "dirty," dishonest process somehow connected with the business world. (Negotiation is used daily, not only when you buy a used car!) Negotiation, when performed effectively, is honest, caring, and nonconfrontational. The success of the process has much more to do with listening carefully and asking questions than with a win or lose argument.

- Remain calm. Separate the person from the problem and avoid seeing the other party as an adversary. The other party is *not* an enemy, but is generally a colleague with whom you must continue to enjoy a positive working relationship. Even if you don't like his or her personality or style, getting along with him or her and negotiating successfully will help you and your department achieve its goals.

- Be patient and plan the timing well. Don't begin negotiations when the situation is not advantageous. Begin negotiating in a neutral territory or, at the very least, on your own turf. Be aware of your own strengths and weaknesses as you plan the negotiations.

- Prior to the meeting, fully explore the worst case scenario. What would happen if you were to come away with the worst of all possible worlds? This will help you determine your bottom line or the worst alternative you'll agree to. Remember that you can always walk away from the negotiations.

- Before negotiations occur, prepare yourself with some objective standards (preferably outside sources) that could be agreed upon as measuring sticks. For example, if your negotiations involve salary, you may wish to do a community survey. If you are insisting on another department to deliver services with a certain degree of quality, locate benchmarking criteria from other facilities.

- Focus on a mutually beneficial outcome for both parties. This is often different from the solution you initially developed, hoping to force this opinion on the other party. Ask, "How will we measure whether we have discovered a mutually beneficial outcome?"

- Think about the other party's needs and position before negotiation, but always ask questions *during* negotiations so that you can fully validate and understand the other person's point of view. Ask, "Help me to see why this is important to you." "If I understand what you are saying, your needs are . . ." Prioritize your own needs, and express these clearly.

- Come up with ideas that allow both parties to have needs met. Stress shared interests and any common ground. When meeting an impasse, reiterate your common ground and your commitment to achieving a positive outcome. Ask the other party, "What would you do if you were in my shoes?"

- Control your emotions. Try to become emotionally divested (as opposed to invested) in the options you like best. Give positive support and empathy for the other party's position as enthusiastically as you support your own needs and position.

- Assess each alternative. Discuss the pros and cons of each and how these would meet each person's needs. Again insist on using objective criteria. Ask "What if?" to discuss alternatives.

- Do not yield to hard bargaining or cajoling; respond only when sound judgment is used. Identify the principles you are using based on logical reasoning. If you feel that you are being pressured, ask, "When you think about the alternative you've come up with, what is it that makes that idea fair, based on our criteria?"

- Whether you use these strategies to bargain for a higher staffing budget or to buy that used car, using a predetermined, planned strategy will put more money in your pocket!

You cannot shake hands with a clenched fist.

Indira Ghandi

REFERENCE

Fisher, R, Ury, W., & Patton, B. (1991). *Getting to yes* (2nd ed.). Boston: Houghton Mifflin Co. Source: GETTING TO YES 2/e, Roger Fisher, William Ury and Bruce Patton. Copyright © 1981, 1991. Houghton Mifflin Co.

SUGGESTED READING

Robbins, A. (1992). *Awaken the giant within.* New York: Simon & Schuster. (Problem solving.)

Weeks, D. (1992). *The eight essential steps to conflict resolution.* New York: Jeremy P. Tarcher, Inc. (Conflict resolution.)

Chapter 11

Why All This Emphasis on Marketing?

A WHILE BACK, we had the opportunity to work with a corporation that had just implemented a major marketing program in all of its health care facilities. At the annual retreat a few months later, the president of the company asked everyone to complete an exercise in which they defined their role within the company. To say he was dismayed when he read the responses from the nursing leaders would be grossly understating his response. His anger and disappointment came from the fact that not one of the nursing staff had listed marketing as part of his or her role. Looking back at the implementation plan it was clear to see that nursing had not been included in any of the planning or presenting (or attending!) of any of the information programs that launched the marketing campaign (oops!).

What's the point here? At the front lines, serving the most important people, nurses are either expected to understand their role in marketing the organization or are overlooked altogether (as in the case above). Lest *you* overlook this very important focus of your role, we have included a few key questions in the following section.

> *Everywhere one sees the growth of a kind of marketing mentality in health care. . . . The "health center" of one era is the "profit center" of the next.*
>
> PAUL STARR

Q #55 The nurse recruiter makes a big deal out of "internal marketing." I'm not even sure what that means. Would you explain?

A You bet. "Internal marketing" is a buzzword that has gained popularity in recent years as health care becomes more and more competitive. Briefly, it refers to all those things you do on the inside of an organization to make certain that the perception on the outside of the organization is as positive as it possibly can be. Satisfying the needs of the internal customers will allow the organization to upgrade its ability to satisfy the external customers. (We know, you are grimacing at the word "customers," but bear with us.) This is, as you have guessed, a complex process that can be better explained with the following points.

- Identify the customer. In the case of internal marketing, these are *your* folks. The employees on the staff (*all* areas) and the physicians as well are the customers of the internal market. It is their needs that must be satisfied in such a manner that they are in turn able to meet the needs of those people who use the facility. Since the doctors are a special group all to themselves, we will discuss their needs (in relation to yours!) in Question 57. For now, let's concentrate on your employees.

- Find out their needs. We talked a lot about this when discussing questions on motivation. Basically, this is the same issue. In a positive, upbeat place where people want to work and are more likely to go the extra mile, employees whose needs have been regarded first felt satisfied. You can't give what you haven't got. (Some nurses have been trying to do this for years!) So take a look at what your staff really needs. We consider some of the following items from Wendy Leebov's (1988) list to be a good place to start:

☐ Economic security—are your employees worried about layoffs, cutbacks, and changes in pay?

☐ Emotional security—do your employees trust management and believe in the mission of the unit?

☐ Recognition—is good work recognized, valued, and appreciated?

☐ Self-expression—is this a "safe" place to share ideas without risk?

☐ A voice in decisions—do staff members feel that they participate in decisions affecting their work?

☐ Access to information—do employees feel they are informed or kept in the dark?

☐ Safety and security—are working conditions satisfactory and safe?

- Assess what your organization is doing to meet these needs. Who better to join you in this assessment than the staff members? Ask them. A quick questionnaire format or a discussion at a staff meeting can give you some clear ideas about how the group feels the organization is doing internally. Take this pulse frequently. And don't wait for the annual survey that human resources might conduct. A monthly update can help you to correct a situation before it gets out of hand. There may be gaps in what staff members perceive and what the organization is actually doing. In your management position, you can often supply information to help clarify misperceptions. A word of advice here (that's what we do!): Take steps to prevent these monthly updates from becoming gripe sessions. Discuss what people need and what they feel they are not getting and ask them to provide realistic solutions. It's no fair complaining without also having a reasonable solution to suggest.

- Put the staff to work. If there are gaps (real or perceived) and morale is down, get your staff members involved in an employee relations committee. This group could take a look at employee needs and what's causing the downward trend in morale and brainstorm options for solutions. If your facility already has such a group, make certain some members of your unit are on it. Do whatever you can to communicate the work of this committee to administration and to the rest of the staff.

- Focus on communication. No matter where we are, there is always someone in the group who says they "are the last to hear about it" or they "never hear it at all." What are you doing to make certain your staff members are in the know when it comes to what's going on in the organization? We know managers who have placed bulletins on mirrors, in the medication room, on time cards, in paychecks, and other creative places. (Recognize your limits—this is often an employee copout—you can and *must* make the information available; but you cannot make them read it!)

- Be open to hearing about problems. When an employee raises an issue about a current policy or practice on your unit, be ready with an open mind. Too often we tend to respond in a way that will turn off all but the most persistent employee. Denying, defending, ignoring, or placating will not endear you in the hearts of your staff. If you have advertised your accessibility and willingness to listen, be prepared to follow through. You may not be able to solve all of your employees' problems. (If you can our hat's off to you!) But you can show them that you respect and value their needs by listening, investigating, and following up with an answer to their concerns.

- Be prepared to go the extra mile. You can't expect your employees to do this if you are not. This does not mean doing their jobs, however. It does mean that you must do everything within your role to make their jobs easier, through improvement of systems, availability of supplies and resources (including staff), and in such a way that each employee feels valued and supported for the contribution he or she makes to the unit. In return, you can expect higher morale and stronger commitment to your unit and to the organization as a whole. Now that's a good return on your investment!

We have forty million reasons. . . but not a single excuse.

RUDYARD KIPLING

Q #56 How do I handle complaints from patients and families?

A Ouch! We all hate to handle complaints because it usually means dealing with unhappy people and it feels like we're not doing our jobs. How much nicer it feels to get that box of candy from the grateful family in room 210! But there are lessons to be learned from complaints and a few strategies for making the process easier.

• Shift your focus. If you approach each complaint with foreboding and feel your personal defenses rising, it's time to change your focus. Look at a complaint not as a personal attack (we know you take these things very personally because that's the nature of caring), but as an opportunity to get things right, a second chance to do it better.

• Use a standard problem solving method. When presented with a complaint, get the facts first, as you would with any problem. This may require some investigation on your part before you are ready to move on to defining the problem. This is an essential step in preventing the tendency to react too quickly (and to string up the guilty party). Once you have the facts and the problem is clear (personal, system, operation, lack of supplies, etc.), consider alternatives for resolution.

- Follow up with the complainer. This is really one of the best forms of external marketing we know. Think about it. When you complain to a service organization about a specific problem, how do you feel when someone actually gets back to you with a response? Our feelings are much more intense when it's health care we're complaining about and not whether the steak ordered was done to perfection. Expectations are higher, and rightly so, as we deal with the primary issues of personal health and well-being. A follow-up letter, a personal phone call, or a visit to the bedside while the patient is still on your unit will make a lasting, positive impression about the quality of care you are providing. Likewise, *not* following up will make an even more lasting negative impression. People do not forget (do you?) and will tell everyone they know about how badly they were treated. If you have time for nothing else, following-up is the essential step that must not be forgotten.

- Enlist your staff in developing a standard of performance or a protocol for patient complaint management. If the unit expectation is consistent and all complaints are handled according to an agreed upon format, you will have gone a long way in the art of complaint management.

- Model the protocol for your staff. Make certain they understand and are able to follow your lead. You cannot always be on the unit, and often complaints will not directly involve you. Empower your staff members to correct troublesome situations by taking action according to your unit protocol. People on the front lines, directly involved in the situations that may be part of the complaint, need to develop skills to handle these potentially difficult moments. By rescuing them or allowing them to turf complaints to you (and they will!), they are being denied an opportunity for development. (They may not welcome this learning opportunity however, and will no doubt expect you to handle all the tough situations!) How do your night shift personnel respond to the patient who is clearly dissatisfied with the nurse assigned to him or her? Do they call the supervisor? Or can they follow the protocol, discuss the problem with the patient, and adjust the assignment if necessary?

- Seek out complaints. Oh no! Do we really mean this? *Yes!* By asking for feedback, you are also sending the powerful message of caring. Follow-up phone calls after discharge can be a very effective way of getting an evaluation of your unit's performance, as well as giving you the personal satisfaction of connection with the patient after he or she has gone home. Make follow-up phone calls a part of your standard of care and have everyone participate. Develop a basic, short list of questions and review (practice) with staff so that everyone is comfortable making these kinds of calls. If you have a patient relations department or a marketing staff, seek their advice and explain your plan.

- Take a look at the patient questionnaires if your facility uses them. (These are survey forms, similar to those you see at top name hotels and restaurants, that ask for your input regarding their service.) What questions are asked on your form? Is nursing measured solely in terms of amenities (friendly, call lights answered promptly, meals served hot, etc.)? If so, consider making sugggestions to revise the form, adding questions that better reflect professional nursing interventions. *Note:* This can be a real opportunity for nursing to decide what the important issues are. For instance, questions regarding understanding of teaching, patient medications, treatments, and diet may be more meaningful and will subtly educate the public to the idea that this is more than just a hotel. The basic public relations questions on room cleanliness, staff friendliness, and the taste of the food are important, but they do not indicate the real reason that the individual was in the facility in the first place. Nursing care, as we all know, is the real reason. But if we continue to only ask questions regarding the amenities of our service, we will continue to be seen more as waitresses and less as the educated professionals that we are. (Oops! We got on a soapbox here!)

Reading an angry letter and listening to an unhappy relative or an irate patient are never easy. You can transform that defensive, uncomfortable feeling into an organized, empowered response that allows you and your staff to make the best of a difficult situation and to learn from it as well.

Almost means not quite. Not quite means not right. Not right means wrong. Wrong means the opportunity to start again and get it right.

DAN ZADRA

Q #57 My marketing director says I need to "market to the physician." What's this all about?

A No doubt about it, the physicians are our customers too. Gone are the days when physicians were on the staff of only one hospital and proclaimed loyalty to that facility for the duration of their practice. As long as physicians control the admitting process and play a key part in determining which facility gets their business, we must market to them to promote *our* facility's business. (This is rapidly changing with the advent of managed care and health care reform but, for now, we would do well to continue the strategies and practices begun in the early seventies. If you find this a little hard to swallow, think of the process as no different than internal marketing for your employees and remember those basic premises. For a quick review, reread Question 55.)

The physicians you work with are a unique group. (We know they think the same about you!) But there are many similarities to their needs and, by understanding them, we have developed a few strategies to make your collaborative efforts a little smoother.

- Involve the doctors. Just as you can't read the minds of your staff members (at least we don't think you can!), don't make assumptions about what the doctors need or would like to see on your unit. You and your staff are here to serve them (yes—in as much as assisting them will make their jobs and yours a little easier) as well as the patients. So *ask* them for input regarding how things are working on your unit.

- Take off the handcuffs! We have heard many a nurse use the excuse that, "I never see that doctor—he always comes in on the evening shift," or "Dr. Smith only covers weekends, so I never get a chance to see him." If Dr. Smith is one of your difficult doctors, causing hassles and grief for the weekend staff, you need to meet with this person. Call and make an appointment to see him or her in the office during the week, or come in on the weekend and meet with the doctor. Likewise, if this is truly a great person and the staff are always singing his or her praises, you will definitely want to make the acquaintance!

- Meet the doctors on their turf. If you're new in your position, and even if you're not, what better strategy than to take a few afternoons and call on all of the doctors who admit to your unit. Stop by their offices for a few moments, business card in hand, and explain your position and your desire to get to know their needs so that you can look forward to a positive working relationship. We guarantee this will have a tremendous impact!

- Ask each doctor to list three pet peeves that really make his or her life difficult. Share these with your staff members so that everyone can work together to make certain these areas are taken care of. Since we believe in fair play, you might consider sharing with this doctor your staff's three pet peeves regarding his or her behavior. An honest commitment from all parties can help to create a positive relationship with even the toughest cookie.

- Get creative. One of the most successful approaches we know involves the idea of spending the day with the physician. This is a real eye opener for many staff members who have the opportunity to see first hand what it feels like for the physician walking onto the unit of a busy facility in the middle of the day. The staff person who accompanies the physician will have a new appreciation for "ease of practice" needs and will also get a chance to observe what other facilities are doing to meet the physician's needs. If the doctor is on the staff of several facilities and has office hours as well, it makes for a very long day that will certainly lead to an empathic understanding of the challenges of the physician's role.

- Review the systems of your unit from the standpoint of a physician. Most doctors are looking for "ease of practice" and will appreciate anything in the system that makes their day and their work a little less stressful. (Don't we all?) What can you do as a manager to make things run smoothly? Are charts where they need to be for clear access? How about test results? X-rays? Someone at the unit to answer questions? Does everyone know the physicians on staff? Do they introduce themselves and offer assistance to the doctor? One chief of staff we know stated that the most impressive unit to him is the one where people are friendly and greet him by name. (It's the little things that usually count, isn't it?)

- Beware of the stereotype. If you are afraid of physicians and expect them all to be ogres (the troll under the bridge) you will get what you expect. By the law of averages alone (the 80/20 rule) *at least* 80 percent of the doctors you work with will be caring, concerned, and willing to work together for smoother practice. *Expect* to find doctors that care and you will. Expect to find resistance and arrogance and you will find that too. It's all what you want to look for and what you are willing to focus on that counts.

> *To make the kind of money most doctors make, you have to see patients every five to ten minutes. You can't sit and chat with them. You can't get to know them as a whole. I also think that when somebody makes as much money as a physician, nobody wants to hear him talking about his pain.*

> ANONYMOUS PHYSICIAN

(from "Doctors Talk About Themselves")

REFERENCE

Leebov, W. (1988). *Service excellence.* Chicago: American Hospital Publishing Co.

Chapter 12

Is It True That Finance Can Be Fun?

WHY SHOULD WE bother about the troublesome money part of health care? The finance issues seem to be a constant topic of conversation: affordable health care, reducing the budget deficit, providing access to those without insurance. Most of us went into health care professions for noble reasons. We wanted to take care of people and help suffering humanity, save lives, and prevent illness, not mess with money issues. We are often too busy at the front lines of health care to worry too much about the bottom line.

However, we *must* attend to the financial part of our jobs for the very reasons we went into health care professions. We are unable to attain our goals for our clients, for our organizations, or for ourselves without an excellent ability to understand and implement a budget. Knowledge of finance, reimbursement, and cost of operations is essential to our empowerment as managers. In this chapter, we've tackled a few of the issues surrounding the "root of all evil" as it relates to the good that we do each day.

Why is there so much month left at the end of the money?

ANONYMOUS

Q #58 No matter what we do, it always comes back to money. How do I negotiate my salary and the salaries of my staff members?

A Your first sentence says it all: We always get around to the money issue, no matter what. Given the complex nature of this question, we're going to tackle your salary first, and apply those principles to any salary negotiation, including the employees you hire. There are two aspects of salary that we want to cover in our answer: the process and the outcomes.

Let's take a look at your position. When you interviewed and were offered this job, several issues were discussed regarding start date, benefits, span of control, title, office space, and, of course, salary. You may have approached the last issue with caution and trepidation, armed with a truckload of advice from your spouse, friends, colleagues, and anyone else you may have sought out for an expert opinion. Such golden truths as "Never ask about money first—they'll think that's all you're interested in," "Don't accept their first offer—they'll think you are desperate," and the final words of wisdom, "Stick to your guns—make them pay you what you're worth" (we suspect this may have come from a well-meaning parent) were freely offered to you.

We have some well-meaning advice of our own that just happens to relate to the process and the outcomes of salary negotiation. Even though you have already lived through this ordeal, you might keep the following in mind the next time you are in a position to negotiate your own salary or when talking to your new hire during an interview.

- Find out what the salary range is for a similar position in other facilities in your area. When getting salary information, ask about the whole package. Often, managers are paid bonuses or incentives in a variety of packages and may have stock options as well. Base salary range may give you a misleading view if you don't get the whole picture.

- Keep a realistic perspective. Sometimes, in the excitement of the interview with the prospect of a promotion, we tend to overlook this very basic strategy. (We have even heard managerial candidates claim they didn't care what they were paid as long as they got the job. This is a great attitude, but one that is seldom lasting as the months wear on and the pressures of the position become a reality.)

- Determine what your bottom line is. Only you can decide this. You must weigh the benefits of the position in terms of what motivates you personally. Salary may not be the primary objective for you, if you consider the promotion and the opportunity to advance in management more important; you will adjust your bottom line accordingly. (Or you may just want an office with a window and will take that at any price!)

- Determine your asking price. Usually, you will be asked what you think you should receive or what your salary requirement is. Many people would rather face a firing squad than be asked this question. "If my price is too high, he will think I am presumptuous; and if it is too low, I will be stuck, and he may wonder why I think so little of myself. And if I hesitate, and have no ready answer, what will the message be?" Ready, aim, fire!

- Plan your approach. Again, this will be dependent on your personal style. We advocate the direct approach, feeling that this is one area where game playing is not a good idea. If this is your first salary negotiation, be honest. Prepare your response to the questions of salary *before* the interview. Practice (preferably not with one of the friends who gave you the advice above!) so that you are comfortable with discussing this important topic. The process of salary negotiation is just as important as the final outcome that is achieved. You will remember *how* the situation occurred, and if the decision was made *fairly*. This will have a significant impact on your working relationship with this new boss. The determination of fairness will be made by both parties; the boss will also be considering your request and how you respond to an offer.

- Anticipate the reaction of the boss. This is not always easy to do, but in planning and practicing your approach, you must consider what you will do if the boss does not accept your initial request and has an offer of his or her own to make. Rather than making an on-the-spot decision, give careful consideration to what alternatives might be suggested and how you would respond.

- Keep it personal. The salary you receive is strictly your business. You and the boss need to be satisfied with both the outcome and how that process transpired. If you feel the process was unfair or that you were taken advantage of, this may color all future interactions with your new boss. On the other hand, if you were both honest and clear about your needs, it could be the beginning of a mutually positive relationship.

Money isn't everything: usually it isn't even enough.

ANONYMOUS

Q #59 The budget: Isn't it a simple case of input and output?

A "So you can't meet for lunch? Oh, I see, it's budget time again. I'll phone you in a month or so." Instead of planning the calendar around holidays and vacations, a manager's time is often dictated by budget deadlines. As much as you may wish to bury financial paperwork under more pleasant tasks, the need to plan the next year's budget and review implementation and variances of the present budget is constant and insistent.

- Re-evaluate your attitude toward finance. Don't become cowed by a chief financial officer who speaks fluent "Financese." Recognize instead that budgeting is really a simple process, not unlike that of maintaining the body's fluid status. If you can measure a human's intake and output, remember that dollars are easier to measure and more precise! If you can balance your checkbook, you can certainly maintain your department's budget, albeit dealing with a higher volume of cash!

  Now, turn to your budget information without fear! We'll examine in more detail the assessment, planning and projection, implementation, and evaluation phases of budgeting.

- Assess past budgets and trends. What do you expect to happen in the future? What technological changes will necessitate capital expenditures or purchase of major equipment? Will you be changing your salary or pay structure as you attempt to reward new competencies and team work? What is expected to happen in union negotiations? Determine the pattern of how well (or poorly) your department has been staying within the budgetary guidelines in the past.

- Plan your programs for the future and project what expenses (both salary and equipment) may be necessary. Talk to other departments/facilities that have attempted similar new programs, and ask about their budget. Will additional computer applications be needed? What is the expected life of the equipment, and will it necessitate increased staff, overtime, or other supplies? How much will it cost to train multiskilled workers? What innovative programs will be needed to recruit and retain staff?

- As you implement the budget, check your revenues (input), and expenses (output). How do the actual numbers compare with the projections you made based on your best guesses and intuition? Be certain to jot down the rationale for variances; it's difficult to remember when you're discussing it with the CEO. For example, in March, we used extra contract staff in order to be ready for the Joint Commission's visit.

- The most challenging and productive component of the budget process is the continual evaluation process. The manager must explain the rationale for the negative budget variances (too much output) and determine why they occurred and if they could have been avoided. It's very possible that your initial projection was inaccurate and based on some faulty data. Or, it's possible that decisions made daily in your department by a supervisor or staff member are adversely impacting your bottom line. (For example, your housekeepers may want to "have an easier weekend" and work with additional staffing. Or your pharmacy technician may be buying a new car and "need the overtime." You may have three nurses on maternity leave, and be paying salary while you pay overtime for replacements.)

- Intervene to impact the budget variances, or adjust your guidelines to fit your actual situation. Flexible budgeting, based on volume, has become the norm in many health care settings. Educate your staff members about the budget and how wise and thrifty decisions will keep everyone happily employed. Keep them informed about their ability to impact the solvency of the organization.

- Although we always encourage thrift (especially in this time of escalating health care expenditures), remember that each dollar spent is *not* coming out of your own pocket. Managers in health care sometimes forgo projects that will truly save money and assure quality care in the future (for example, staff education) because of an initial cash outlay. Investing in human beings certainly reaps more enduring rewards than playing the stock market!

Economists are people who work with numbers but who don't have the personality to be accountants.

ANONYMOUS

Q #60 Do you have any creative strategies for cutting the budget?

A You've worked painstakingly to come up with an honest, thrifty budget. You've adopted a "no fat" attitude for your department. And then, the dictum comes down from on high: "There's going to be another budget cut of 10 percent across the board!" You're wondering if Marie Antoinette felt this way when she trudged to the guillotine. "But I never *told* them to eat cake; our budget has been on a bread and water basis for years!"

Reactivity rather than proactivity during a time of budget crisis and cuts may not only cost staff jobs, but may cost you your own. Handle with care!

• Obtain more specific information about the extent of the budget cuts. Determine why the budget is being cut, and whether the "across the board" slash treats the real causes of the problem. Is there room for negotiation?

• Determine your department's value and contribution to the overall goals of the organization. Are you performing essential support or other services? Be aware how budget cuts may impact the total service you are attempting to provide, and document the possible effects of the intended cut.

• Meet with staff members and explain the truth about the budget crisis. If you think they haven't heard, you haven't had experience with the efficiency of the grapevine. Quell rumors and fears with as many facts as you may have. Assure them about the process and that you'll keep them informed. If they can be involved in the planning or in coming up with cost-saving ideas, encourage them to work together as soon as possible. They'll certainly be motivated to find alternatives to staffing cuts.

- Be certain that unions are informed from the outset. They'll need to be brought into the decision making early, rather than be in a position to react negatively after cuts are made.

- Establish a plan and timeline for decreasing the budget while maintaining service levels. Whatever creative ideas you may develop, don't lay off staff precipitously. Often, this will cost you more in terms of turnover, orientation, abuse of sick leave, and loss of productivity.

- Take time to make the necessary changes *correctly*. Be certain that you have engaged in a thorough assessment and planning process prior to making recommendations for further budget cuts. Hasty decisions without adequate planning always end up costing more money than is saved.

- Be creative. Sometimes the impetus of a budget crisis encourages us to stretch ourselves and our systems beyond the norm to come up with even better methods of serving our clients. (Do you need to change care delivery systems? Can you use short-term contract workers? How can downtime in one department be used as person power in another?)

- Attempt to avoid competition and resentment among departments. (Why was he allowed to retain all of his staffing budget while I had to decrease mine by 30 percent? Who does he know that I don't?) Competing for scarce resources often puts managers in adversarial positions. Try to support and help each other, looking together at the bigger organizational financial picture for potential savings.

There was a time when a fool and his money were soon parted, but now it happens to everybody.

ADLAI STEVENSON

REFERENCE

Hansten, R. & Washburn, M. (1992, October). The budget cut nightmare—How to keep it from happening to you. *Aspen's Advisor for Nurse Executives.* Gaithersburg, MD: Aspen Publishers, Inc. [newsletter].

Chapter 13

How Can We Survive and Still Deliver Quality Nursing Care?

AS MUCH AS we'd like to avoid them, the basic issues of staffing, scheduling, and creating care delivery systems despite environmental challenges tend to require a huge amount of our time as nurse managers. We could immerse ourselves in all the most rewarding and enjoyable activities in management if only our fairy godparent would flick his or her magic wand over our units and—poof! there would be the right number (not too many, not too few!) and type (productive, motivated, and well-trained) of skilled personnel to take the very best care of our patients.

Although we'd like to act as fairy godmothers, we can't produce this fantasy land for you. Here are some hints on how to contend with staffing/scheduling, care delivery systems, and the issue of nurse assistive personnel. You'll have to adapt our ideas to your own situation.

Buck up! These issues can be time-consuming and even frustrating. They are also basic to the functioning of your unit and essential to your ability to move toward your vision. Once these building blocks are in place, you're ready for any new challenge!

> *I have never been as resigned to ready-made ideas as I was to ready-made clothes, perhaps because although I couldn't sew, I could think.*

> JANE RULE

Q #61 Are there any easier methods for staffing and scheduling?

A We're not here to tell you how to count bodies or hours or the formula for full time equivalent employees and patient care hours. Those issues don't really seem to be the most problematical, do they? When there's a shortage of personnel in your region, or if you are managing a "difficult" service, finding enough of the right people to do the work is a constant headache. At times, dealing with illness, work-related injuries, leaves of absence, and night shift coverage can be so time-consuming that your other work and favorite projects become lost in the shuffle. When you've made so many calls pleading for extra shifts that your ear begins to conform to the shape of the telephone receiver, you know it's time to try new strategies.

Having the appropriate number of staff members available is a number one priority. It's difficult to coach a high performance team on to higher and higher levels of quality without enough players on the team. It is worth it, however, to streamline the process so that the team can deliver that quality care.

- If you have had difficulty recruiting your staff, it's time to think about how you market your department internally and externally. You need a new image, and your staff members will be the best people to help you create it. (See Chapter 11.)

- Staffing is closely related to the budget. Be creative about how to use those employees within your budget guidelines. Despite the rituals and rules we tend to have in nursing regarding shift hours and types of care delivery systems, think about being creative with different shifts and different types of workers, when using the money you do have.

- While you think of creative new solutions, also maintain flexibility. Staffing and scheduling flexibility are among the most commonly discussed "job satisfiers" for nurses, and will continue to be expected by the workers of the future. Can shifts and days off be modified? Are people able to attend to family situations (within reason)?

- Decide whether your staff is ready to do self-scheduling, and plan to implement the system. Although it may take some time to train and oversee the process at first, your employees will gain understanding of the situations you've been encountering. This staff accountability will encourage further professional growth and will ease your burden! You move out of the "mom" or "dad" role and expect employees to be accountable for their work time. If possible, delegate phone calls and other pieces of scheduling if your staff members aren't yet ready to do it all themselves.

- As your staff members redesign shifts or care delivery, ask the librarian to do a literature search. Some schedules have worked better than others, depending on the clinical area and organization. Be on the lookout for the following pitfalls:

  ☐ Does this new shift create other budget drains, such as increased overtime, difficulty in relief coverage, or loss of productivity during the final hours of the shift?

  ☐ How will reporting be done accurately between shifts? This is especially difficult with combinations of shift hours, but can be accomplished.

  ☐ Who is supervising the assistive personnel?

  ☐ On overlapping shifts, is the work you'd intended being completed? Are individual work style variances affecting this? (An energetic and efficient worker will be able to make any shift work, while those with less initiative and a slower pace may not.)

- Despite the challenges of dealing with overtime or compensatory time, many of the positions in your organization may adapt to a salary concept. (Dare we say it? Are we professionals or not? Salaries are a significant reflection of the professional services we render.)

- Especially if your unit has wide variance in census, you won't always be able to exactly predict your staffing needs. If you've overstaffed, you'll severely impact the budget. (Somehow we think you already know this!) Within union regulations or other policies, encourage flexibility for staff members to leave early or take a vacation day if census is low. If, on the other hand, patients are overly abundant, find a way to provide additional staff members through float pools or on-call staff rather than using more expensive agency assistance.

- Staffing and scheduling are other areas of your job in which you don't have all the control you'd want. You can't control the acuity of the patients, the health and wellness of your staff members and their families, or other unforeseen circumstances. Be certain you've done all you can, that you've instituted staffing support processes as discussed above, and then be at peace.

Reality is something you rise above.

LIZA MINELLI

Q #62 Should I change the care delivery system in my department?

A What's it going to be? Primary care, case management, patient focused care, teams, or modular nursing? Strawberry, chocolate cheesecake, neopolitan, or nonfat yogurt? Choose a new flavor and you'll soon hear your staff saying,

"Well, they are making another change in the care delivery system! The pendulum swings one way and then the other. Years ago we had a staff of RNs, LPNs, and nursing assistants. Then an 'all RN' staff and total patient care was in vogue. Now we can't afford all RNs, and we're going back to nursing assistants! When can we just do our jobs without all these changes in the way we do our care!?"

Many of us would agree: We've been in nursing for a couple of decades, and we've seen every type of care delivery system tried for one reason or another. It doesn't seem like you're keeping up with the latest trends if you don't adopt the most recent fad. Yet, as a manager who must deliver the highest quality care with limited human and budgetary resources, a change of the methods by which care is given may achieve the best utilization of available personnel. In this age of health care reform, *creativity may equal survival*. How does a manager decide?

- Determine the characteristics of an *optimal* care delivery system. Decide what kinds and quantities of patients need care, within which levels of quality and by which standards. How would all personnel be utilized? Refer to your mission and vision.

- Think about which parts of the current care delivery system work well and should be preserved. For example, if RNs are able to supervise other personnel while they coordinate care with other disciplines, write that down as a non-negotiable constant.

- Decide which aspects of the current care delivery system aren't working as well as could be expected. Do the nursing assistants have downtime with nothing to do? Are the RNs overburdened with heavy lifting and other patient care duties without help? Is there confusion on the part of physicians about who is taking care of whom?

- Record your "givens" in terms of budget, personnel resources, educational systems, types of care being delivered.
Once you've recorded these givens, challenge them. If any of
these are stumbling blocks, think about creative methods of
changing them. For example, if your personnel budget
seems too low for the required level of staffing coverage,
plan to reallocate financial resources based on potential revenue. Or consider how to deliver the same "amount" of care
less expensively. Think about other ways of educating staff
to fill different roles if your educational department isn't
able to help you out. Can your unit add a service of less acute
patients to the current complement and spread the acuity
differently? If you need further numbers of staff for desk
coverage, would two nurse assistive personnel equal one
tenured RN salary, or would one secretary do the job?

- Think now about the details of what goes on during each
shift on your unit. *Now* is the time to *be there* on each shift,
and on weekends, to observe and ask questions. Meet with
staff members or put together task forces that answer the following questions:

  ☐ Which tasks or processes aren't being done as well as
  you'd like them to be? (Look at unusual occurrence reports, errors, complaints, staff input.)

  ☐ Which staff are doing tasks that someone else could/
  should do? Do any of the job descriptions contain overlapping functions?

  ☐ How are people rewarded and for what behaviors? Does
  talking together at the desk seem to be more rewarding
  than charting assessments? Are tasks being seen as most
  important, with long-term planning for the patients coming up third or lower in the priority list?

  ☐ What duties are occupying the nurses' time? What about
  the time of each of the other personnel?

☐ Look into the details of your department as they relate to the type of patient: Do the respiratory therapists (if you are lucky enough to have them) make rounds at certain times and wait with a cup of coffee while the treatments are being done? Is chemotherapy spaced throughout the shift or is it heavier from 4:00 to 8:00 P.M.? What happens on each shift will help determine the work flow and need for overlap or different types of personnel.

☐ Whom do you want to manage the patient throughout his care? Will it be a primary nurse, a case manager, or whoever happens to get assigned to the patient during the next few shifts? Determine how you want professional nursing to best influence the outcomes of the patient and to coordinate the care.

☐ How will physicians, nurses, and other health care professionals communicate? Will you use rounds, communication sheets, the chart forms, or multiple phone calls?

☐ Determine the transport issue within your organization. Who transports supplies, people, equipment, mail? Some facilities are beginning to use robots for some of these. If you can't find a warm body, use a cold one.

☐ Who is best able to provide cleaning and other environmental services?

☐ What specifics in technology affect your service and the care delivery?

☐ Find several tasks that can be eliminated and duplication that can become a single effort. What work is more efficient using two people? Come up with prizes for staff members who develop methods of eliminating duplication.

• Collect and review articles about different care delivery systems to further enhance your creativity; telephone those facilities that have tried new ideas and get the real story from them. Be certain that staff members are involved in this exploration as well and that you talk to those on the front line that are truly experiencing the system.

- Don't duplicate a plan from a workshop or article and decide it's the perfect system for you. *Any care delivery system must be adapted to your own organization and department.* Change only those things that need to be changed, and be sure you can articulate a good reason for doing so.

- Your care delivery system framework, whether you adopt a specific nursing theory or use common sense, must reflect you and your staff's philosophy of the role of professional nursing. Whatever flavor you choose, make an informed choice!

> *Nurses must recognize that the traditional frameworks within which nursing care is practiced are no longer adequate to the needs of the consumer, nor are they adequate to the current practice environment. This is the first step in beginning to deal with some of the major changes that will be driving health care well into the twenty-first century.*
>
> TIM PORTER-O'GRADY

Q #63 How can we avoid the "Frankenstein Syndrome" as we use multiskilled workers and other nurse extenders?

A As you explore new care delivery systems and read current literature, you'll see a trend that pairs registered nurses with other types of workers. Some of these workers' job descriptions include hybrid combinations of several of the more conventional roles. We've seen combinations of respiratory therapists, phlebotomists, nursing assistants, emergency medical technicians, and medical assistants. In orthopedic services, a physical therapy assistant may be trained to do nursing assistant work as well as some secretarial duties. These multiskilled assistants often work extremely well in delivering high quality patient care; plus they keep valuable and talented people employed during rough financial times.

We'd all agree that creativity is essential in encouraging all personnel to become their most productive in today's health care environment. However, as much as this creativity may ensure survival of your organization, be certain you follow these steps so that your redesigned roles and multiskilled workers don't become facility Frankensteins! Poorly planned personnel changes are not only painful to the employee (who trusted you and even adapted!), but can become nightmares if you've interpreted state regulations improperly.

- Take a look at the tasks now being performed by registered nurses. Which tasks could be given away to someone else while preserving the RN's ability to supervise and be accountable?

- Determine which basic skills are needed for the type of service you provide. For example, if you manage a respiratory area, respiratory therapy skills may make the best basis for cross training. If you are working in a skilled nursing facility, you may wish to cross train a combination of workers, such as physical therapy aids, nursing assistants, or other therapists.

- *Reread your state nurse practice act!* Find out what certification and/or licensure is needed for all the duties you'd like performed. Whether you have questions or not, call your state licensing board and talk about your ideas. Many states are now wrestling with some of these issues and changes in state policy will be occurring. Be certain you do not ask staff members to perform procedures for which they are not trained or certified. Be certain they do not independently take on duties beyond their revised job descriptions. (Here's where the nightmare potential is very grim!)

- Before you embark on a training program, assess your nursing staff's ability to delegate clinical skills and remain accountable for the nursing care of the patient. Clinical delegation skills may seem simple and basic to you as a manager, but don't assume nurses have been taught how to supervise assistive personnel. We can tell you honestly from traveling throughout the United States teaching this skill, many nurses have not mastered the delegation process. *The ability to delegate appropriately and supervise staff effectively so that the registered nurse can comfortably remain accountable for high quality patient care is essential to the success of any care delivery system (or creative assistive personnel roles) you create.* Attention to this point is much more effective than wearing a clove of garlic or keeping a drawer full of silver bullets.

- As you and your staff are developing the roles for your multiskilled assistive personnel, keep asking the assistants, as well as your RN staff, hard questions about the plan. They will have the best idea of how well the changes will work. (As you listen, sift out the negative talk of those who resist change no matter what! Focus them on the benefits they'll enjoy if they work to make this happen!)

- Before the roles change, hold staff meetings that include a discussion of each new worker's job description. Ask staff: "What will you expect a nursing care assistant to do? What will the NCAs expect the RNs to do?" Ask about tasks, but also about such fine points as, "Whose responsibility is it to answer call lights? Answer the phone? Talk to the doctors, families, or other health care workers?" Even though you should expect conflict to increase when changes occur, role ambiguity will cause more conflict than you'd care to imagine and has the potential for harming patients. Another potential thriller!

- *Be there for implementation!* As ill-advised as it may seem, time and time again we see managers staying away from the first shifts when their department is starting a new system. Put all your other work on hold. If you aren't there to lend support and work on glitches, all your preparation may be in vain. (Each shift may seem like Halloween, but you'll be there with your staff to be sure the treats don't become tricks!)

- After the new assistive personnel have been working in your department for several weeks, hold additional meetings to again discuss their roles and clarify questions. Ask each group to identify, "What do you wish your RN understood about your job as a patient care assistant?" and vice versa. Again clarify what each group expects of the other regarding duties, communication, and methods of feedback and supervision.

- Recognize that RNs' supervision of other personnel will encourage them to learn new management skills. Be certain that the required education is forthcoming for all groups. From our experience, we've noted that training and practice in assertive communication, conflict resolution, giving feedback, and evaluation techniques are essential.

- At the six month point, the roles and workers should have synergized. Continue support in terms of education, evaluation of the system, and listening to staff. But this is also time to celebrate your hard work: You haven't created a monstrous nightmare. Instead you've facilitated a process that has empowered all your staff members to grow as they deliver patient care effectively and efficiently. You'll all be ready for one night's restful sleep before the next challenge hits!

> *I never did anything worth doing by accident; nor did any of my inventions come by accident; they came by work.*
>
> THOMAS EDISON

Chapter 14

How Do I Avoid Being Bored with the Boards?

THE MENTION OF a board meeting of any nature generally brings a yawn or two. An image of important people sitting around a table, looking official, and talking endlessly about amazingly small details does suggest boredom. But, lest you succumb to that sleepy notion, we have created the following section to address the most important aspects of two of the primary regulatory agencies in your professional life: the state board of nursing and the organizational board at your facility. (No, we have NOT forgotten the Joint Commission—how could we? However, it performs a role all its own, and questions on the Joint Commission are covered in Chapter 15.)

We were going to ask you why you think you should know about these boards. But we've decided you already know. As a manager, one of your many duties is that of policy enforcement. As *successful* managers of our profession's future, we encourage not only a working knowledge of your governing boards, but an active participation as well. Would you let an architect design your house without any input from you? We think not. Why not help to shape the policies and the mission that you will enforce?

> *We are all held in place by the pressure of the crowd around us. We must all lean upon others. Let us see that we lean gracefully and freely and acknowledge their support.*

> MARGARET COLLIER GRAHAM

Q #64 The governing board of my facility is beyond me. That's an executive level I don't feel qualified (or comfortable) to join, and my administration feels the same. Why not let the board do its job and I'll do mine?

A You ask some provocative questions that are not always easy to answer! If you are early in your management career, this "hands off" position is understandable. It's enough to grasp your own role without tackling the big folks at the top. But at some point we suggest that you will seek a better understanding of your organizational board and perhaps consider active involvement as well. Remember, involvement can be attained in a number of ways. Calling a member of the board to simply introduce yourself and describe the work on your unit is a way of being involved. The degree of involvement will certainly be your choice, as this group will function without you! The motivation leading to your action will no doubt dictate the approach you take. For instance, if the board has ruled that the physicians on staff will be exempt or protected from the verbal abuse policy recently drafted by nursing administration (never happens, right?), you may feel a real desire to get to know this group and find out the rationale for its decision. Before you jump into a board meeting, loaded for action, STOP! Consider the following steps:

• Start with your nurse executive. A meeting with this individual is a good way to begin to understand the organizational makeup of the board—who the members are (is the nurse executive one?) and what the role of this group is (real and perceived) within your organization.

There are a variety of functions possible for an executive board, based on the size and nature of your facility. Hospital boards may truly be governing bodies, with representation from medical staff, administration, and the community at large. Or their primary interest may be the protection of the stockholders' interests, which will be accomplished in part by the assurance that management is keeping things running smoothly in a profitable direction.

Explain to the nurse executive your interest in understanding the total picture of the organizational framework of your facility: the nature of the board, when it meets, who attends, and what it does, are good places to start.

- Attend a board meeting. First find out if these meetings are open for general attendance (usually they are, but check it out to make sure). Again, your nurse executive may be able to assist by making it possible for you to attend as a guest, and perhaps to share with the board an overview of the area that you manage. (In some cases, this is a very radical request and will not be warmly received. Yet we've worked with other organizations in which inviting department managers to give brief reports to the board is an expected practice!)

- Obtain copies of the minutes of the board meetings. If attendance is not encouraged, or denied altogether, see if you can get copies of meeting minutes so that you can have an overview of the actions of this group. You might want to also know why these meetings are closed. Does this say something about your organizational culture?

- Get to know the board members. This a form of political strategy (see Question 15 on power and politics for a refresher) as well as one of internal marketing (Question 55). A word of emphasis and encouragement is necessary here: There is nothing stopping you from forming relationships with these individuals who play an important part in shaping the direction of the facility for which you work. Take off those mental handcuffs that tell you that this is something you can't (or shouldn't) do because no other manager is doing it. Talk to the physicians on the board, talk to the community members, talk to administration—in a positive and informative way. (No whining!) Sharing what you do and the insights you and your staff have from working directly on the front lines will help the board members to be more informed. And, as we all know, clearer decisions are made when there is more information.

Bad administration, to be sure, can destroy good policy; but good administration can never save bad policy.

ADLAI STEVENSON

Q #65 What should I know about the board of nursing? They're on my side, aren't they?

A This is a great question—we're glad you asked! It's always amazing to us that so few practicing professional nurses are truly aware of the board of nursing and its functions. It's as if the existence of this regulatory body is accepted, but acknowledged only when we renew our license or, horror of horrors, are called by the board to respond to a complaint. That, dear friends, is *not* the time to get to know this important agency. Instead, we are in favor of a more proactive approach and will therefore spend the next few moments providing a brief overview of some key aspects of the board.

- What is the primary duty of the board? Like any state regulatory agency, the primary duty of the board of nursing in any state is to protect the safety of the public. This is accomplished through the many functions that you may be aware of: regulation of licensure, investigation of complaints, review of schools providing nursing education, monitoring of the licensure exam, and revision and enforcement of your state's nurse practice act.

- Who are the members of the board? Again, this is a state agency, and the members are selected through a government appointment process that varies from state to state. The size of the board, the term of office for each member, and the type of membership representation are outlined in your state practice act. Generally, there will be representation of the major categories of practice (education, community health, maternal/child, general clinical, and one lay person).

- What is the difference between the staff of the board and the board members? There are usually support personnel hired by the agency to provide administrative, clerical, and consultant (or investigative) support to the board. These are employees of the board, not members who participate in the decision-making processes of the board itself. A consultant may call you to investigate a complaint made to the board, but the board members will receive the report and make the decisions regarding the final ruling on the complaint.

- What is the source of authority for the board of nursing? We know you know the answer to this question. In fact, we bet you even keep a copy of it by your bed for late night reading! Seriously, the answer is the nursing practice act, which is the legislated law that describes the scope of nursing practice within your state. If you don't have a copy, both in your office and available to the staff, we encourage you to get one soon. This document will outline the board, its membership, staff, and duties, as well as address key practice issues that you as a manager and a nurse must know.

- Are there boards in every state? Yes. This is a government agency that you can't escape! The size and structure of the board itself may vary from state to state, but the primary duties will remain the same. For instance, in Washington and California, there are separate boards for registered nurses and licensed practical nurses, while in Arizona, RN and LPN practices are regulated by the same board. In recent years, the certification of nursing assistants and monitoring of unlicensed assistive personnel has also been added to the duties of many of the state boards of nursing. All nursing boards from each state send representation to the National Council of State Boards of Nursing. This group meets regularly to strive for national standardization of practice and to address global issues that are applicable to nursing practice, no matter what the region.

• Can I call the board of nursing? Absolutely! This agency is in existence to protect the public (that's you!) by regulation of the state's nurse practice act (again, that's you). We strongly recommend that you develop a working relationship with the members of this group, one that goes beyond that phone call to check on the licensure status of a new hire. There may be a time when you will be more involved with this agency, either by choice or through an investigatory process of one of your staff members or yourself. The time to understand the duties of the board is before you are placed in one of these situations. We refer you to the next series of questions for more strategies for building positive relationships with the members of the board. Read on!

> *For is it not that human progress is but a mighty growing pattern woven together by the tenuous single threads united in a common effort?*
>
> MADAME CHIANG KAI-SHEK

Q #66 Clear something up for me, please. You recommend knowing the nurse practice act and contacting the board of nursing for assistance, but everything seems so vague. How do I get a straight answer to my questions?

A This can be one of the more frustrating aspects of your managerial role. It is true that most nurse practice acts are not specific laundry lists that spell out in black and white what truly is and is not the practice of nursing. The generic approach allows for the flexibility of the law to adapt to the profession as it changes and grows. We suspect that most nurses would take exception to the confining nature of a specific list of tasks as their practice act. A more general approach requires interpretation, yes, but also allows us to practice the critical thinking component of our profession and not just focus on a series of described tasks. The list would be easier to evaluate and more comfortable to apply, but where's the art of nursing?

Now that you are thoroughly frustrated and realize that this is not the straight answer you requested, let's take a look at some of the specific resources you have available to assist you in the interpretation of the legal aspect of your job.

- *Rules and/or regulations.* Generally, the nurse practice act is supplemented by another document that may be referred to as the "rules and regs," the regulatory code, or simply "the rules." This document will add more specific descriptions to what is generically stated in the act itself. Without going into a lot of detail on the political/legislative processes, we suggest that when you contact the board to inquire about meetings, you also find out what the legal documents are that govern your practice in your state. You may find the specific rules to be a little easier to follow. It is in this document that you are more likely to find a "list" format and more clearly outlined details of practice parameters. One list you will certainly find is that of "unprofessional conduct" (commonly referred to as "what you can do that will get you into trouble," this is one area that lends itself easily to the list format).

- *Impaired nurse or diversion program.* This program may be legislated in the practice act and more completely defined in the rules portion. In recent years, nursing boards have taken a proactive stance rather than their original punitive approaches when dealing with a nurse who is involved in substance abuse. Knowing this program and the expectations of you as a nursing manager will assist you when faced with the difficult situation of an employee who is abusing drugs. Do you know what you should do if a nurse you hire states she is on the diversion program? And are you clear about the actions required if you suspect an employee is impaired? These are tough questions, with straight answers that are available to you through the program established by your board. (Of course, your facility will have policies as well, and we are not suggesting that these be overlooked!)

- *Advisory opinions.* We'll discuss committees in the next question. (The ones that you have no time for, but that one of your staff members might be just the right candidate for!) Well, those committees will sometimes be called upon to interpret a part of the practice act or the rules that may be particularly confusing or controversial. In those cases, a committee may study the situation and develop an "advisory opinion," which will address the issue in greater detail and apply it to practice. Once approved by the board, these opinions are available for reference and will help to clarify a sometimes confusing situation. For example, the issue of abandonment may be confusing in your current practice act and may not be clearly spelled out in specific terms. What qualifies as abandonment? If a nurse reports to duty and refuses her assignment on the basis of safety (not enough staff to provide safe care), is she guilty of abandonment of her patients? An advisory opinion would assist in the interpretation of this definition as it applies to your practice. If the question comes up often enough to the board (and we suspect that this one does), an advisory opinion will be created and/or the act will be revised when possible.

- *The board members.* As we said earlier, these folks are appointed by the governor to protect the public through the regulation of nursing practice. They write the rules, set the standards, and interpret the law as it applies to nursing practice. They are, or can be, a pretty powerful group! Make use of their expertise and positions!

One of the most heartfelt cries you will hear from your staff members will be the statement (made with considerable emotion: anger, determination, and fear are good ones!), "I'm not putting *my* license on the line!" When faced with this situation, you will want to be able to respond with confidence and authority as you clarify for the nurse just what legal risks she is taking. If you are not certain yourself, then we recommend speaking directly to a member of the board for clarification. A note of advice here: Correspondence of this type is fairly important, so you will certainly want to put it in writing. Call, for more immediate feedback, and then send a letter to follow up. This will establish that ever important paper trail of documentation. We suggest this form of action whether you speak to a staff person at the board or a board member.

Be patient. You are dealing with a state agency, and some things will take time, based on the complexity of the question. What you perceive to be a simple question may be subject to interpretation by the entire board and even the attorney general. Straight answers are not always immediately available, but you must be willing to persist, establish a trail of documentation, and become knowledgeable about the process. It's *your* practice!

The feeble tremble before opinion, the foolish defy it, the wise judge it, the skillful direct it.

Manon Roland

Q #67 What can the board of nursing do for me?

A When you were a staff nurse, you probably had little interaction with the board of nursing, other than to renew your
license or to read the periodic newsletter that they might
publish. Moving to a new state, you became aware of the
requirements of that particular agency and may have noted
differences in continuing educational classes and the fees
charged for a new license. Beyond these obvious functions,
you probably became more aware of other benefits the
board provides when you assumed your management position. Hiring personnel generally means a phone call to
check on licensure status, and if one of your staff does not
perform within the limits of the practice act, you may also
get to know the board very quickly. Is there anything else
beyond discipline and regulation that you should know
about? (Hey—who's asking the questions here?)

As we mentioned in the previous question, we believe
strongly in the idea of building a working relationship with the
members of this agency. Of course, relationships are best when
they are two-sided. John Kennedy's famous statement can be
paraphrased here as, "Ask not what your board can do for you,
ask what you can do for your board." Here then, are some basic
ideas for you to consider when getting to know the board of
nursing in your state.

• Attend a board meeting. With the exception of an executive
  session, all meetings are posted and open to the public. A
  phone call to the board will get you a list of its scheduled
  meetings, and the agenda for the next meeting. Explain to
  the staff person that you are interested in learning more
  about the agency and its functions and will be attending a
  meeting in the future. There may be informational literature
  that can be sent to you as well, to help you prepare for what
  you will be observing. Board meetings are usually one or

two full days, depending on the amount of business to be covered, and are typically held monthly or bimonthly. Some states even rotate their meeting sites around the state to give people an opportunity to attend without having to travel too far.

- Speak to a consultant or the executive director of the board about the possibility of a staff member or a board member visiting your facility to meet with your staff to describe the duties and activities of the board. Your staff development person may also be involved in planning this "Board 101" presentation. We're willing to bet that the majority of your staff members do not have a clear idea of the function of this group, yet they willingly write annual checks to cover the costs of a nursing license. Planning an informational session will have many positive effects—and will certainly let the board know that you are interested in what they are doing on your behalf.

- When planning a change in care delivery, a change in the traditional job roles on your unit, or an expansion of a current role, contact the board for input. Many of the creative delivery approaches being used today have the potential for asking someone to practice nursing without a license. The consultant staff can assist you in making certain that what you are proposing is not restricted by your practice act.

- Volunteer for a committee. Knowing how busy you are, we make this suggestion carefully (you may want to send us hate mail). Short of an appointment to the board by the governor (which is not a bad position to consider sometime in your career), this is one of the best ways to become involved in shaping the regulation of nursing in your state. Most boards use the committee process to encourage participation of practicing professionals in developing new revisions to the practice act or assisting in interpretations of current law.

Volunteers are appointed by the board for various committees based on the particular area of expertise and experience
of the individual. If you do not feel you have the time for this
commitment, consider developing one of your staff members by supporting them in volunteering. A scope of practice
committee, legislative affairs committee, or one of the other
committees may be the perfect fit for one of your employees
who is looking for an opportunity to become more professionally involved. What better way as a manager to facilitate
professional growth and to assist the board at the same time!

*Never doubt that a small group of thoughtful, committed
citizens can change the world. Indeed, it is the only thing
that ever has.*

MARGARET MEAD

Chapter 15

Are All These Acronyms Important?

THE JOINT COMMISSION on Accreditation of Healthcare Organizations (JCAHO) is your friend. Or so you've been told. (Why then are other managers dithering in a high anxiety state for six months before the Joint Commission's onsite visit?) And it's true, isn't it, that continuous quality improvement (CQI) or total quality management (TQM) (or other quality initiatives) will improve patient care? (Then explain why some managers still groan when the "Q-words" are mentioned?)

Frankly, it's difficult to identify the supportive and friendly nature of organizations and processes that use acronyms instead of easily understood names! During weaker or more frustrated moments, you may think of the Joint Commission as "Big Brother watching" or quality initiatives as the mind control of some evil-intentioned computer from a science fiction thriller. Lest paranoia set in, let's take the time to get to know these acronyms on a first name basis!

Confusion is a word we have invented for an order which is not understood.

HENRY MILLER

Q #68 Another manager told me my job could be on the line if my unit didn't meet the Joint Commission standards. What should I do to prepare for the surveyors' visit?

A As a new manager, you may still be a bit confused (and afraid to ask) about the role of the Joint Commission (or other accrediting agencies, depending on your type of service). As you understand its role in your life, you'll be apt to see a Joint Commission visit less as an attack from Attila the Hun and more as a benevolent white knight encouraging and assisting your organization to remain viable in the midst of health care chaos.

• Understand the origin and development of the Joint Commission, and then help your staff members understand it as well. It developed as a byproduct of the need to standardize hospitals and surgery and was formed in 1952 by the American Medical Association, American Hospital Association, American College of Physicians, and American College of Surgeons (Roberts, Coale, and Redman, 1987). Still voluntary (your organization pays for the onsite visit and recommendations), health care organizations value the Joint Commission's accreditation for many reasons: good reputation, licensure for Medicare and Medicaid reimbursement (you need accreditation for public funding revenue!), and to fulfill the need for expert evaluation and advice for quality improvement.

• Read (or at least scan) the most recent Joint Commission manual. There will be specific standards that relate to your responsibilities and your area. If you have questions or are daunted by the sheer volume of material, ask your supervisor for assistance. Many facilities keep a standards checklist to assist managers in preparation. If your organization doesn't yet have one, you may wish to design one for yourself. If you plan on staying in this managerial role, you'll need it again!

- Review your department's ability to meet the standards. At a minimum, you and your staff should understand the following:

  - ☐ Staff members (and the manager) should be able to document or point out visible evidence of an interdisciplinary team approach to quality assessment and improvement.

  - ☐ The Joint Commission will expect that your patient and staff safety plan is complete, with up to date documentation.

  - ☐ Review and be in compliance with department standards, policies, and procedures.

  - ☐ Pay close attention to your documentation on patient charts; have clear documentation of staff competencies and/or skills and training.

  - ☐ Keep licensure, accreditation, and certification records up to date for all personnel in your department.

- Be aware of the changes expected as the Joint Commission implements its Agenda for Change. Your surveyors will be emphasizing actual clinical involvement and outcome-oriented monitoring and evaluation in the improvement of patient care quality. This means they will actually be going into the rooms, talking with patients, and asking questions of staff members.

- As you work with the surveyor during a site visit, don't use him or her as a way of placing blame on other departments or of calling attention to a specific shortcoming (your favorite ax to grind). Be honest but open to suggestions.

- Feel free to ask questions and to point out your department's achievements. After all, you are paying for the evaluation and for expert advice.

- Look at this as an opportunity for positive feedback! There's no better way to show your supervisor and your staff members what a wonderful job you've all been doing the last months or years than with a great Joint Commission onsite visit. Enjoy the appreciation and accolades! Now don't you feel that you could be on a first name basis with the Joint Commission? ("Hey, Joi, what about a cup of coffee to celebrate?")

> **Robin:** *Batgirl! What took you so long?* **Batgirl:** *You wouldn't believe the traffic, and the lights were all against me. Besides, you wouldn't want me to speed, would you?* **Robin:** *Your good driving habits almost cost us our lives!* **Batman:** *No, Robin, she's right. Rules are rules.*

Q #69 QA, CQI, TQM: What's the difference?

A Many, many years ago, in a land far, far away, health care managers groaned at the thought of doing still more chart audits that would only, once again, display evidence that some staff members weren't performing according to standard. They knew they had little control or influence over the more global systems affecting their staff's ability to meet standards; nor was it an easy task to attempt to work with the other disciplines affecting their patients' care. Often, the audit data were used against the manager for reprimand. (How motivating!) Yes, quality "assurance" implied a state of ongoing perfection that was in truth often an exercise in managerial frustration.

Have the above circumstances changed in your facility? Certainly, we as managers always believed that quality patient care was (and remains) our fundamental mission. But through the new quality initiatives, we can now hope for fundamental systems overhaul and interdisciplinary teamwork that may encourage us to continually strive for better quality care. (As you read, see if any of our tried and true nursing methods fit here!)

- Review the quality program as it has been set up in your organization. Although organizations may adopt the ideas of one quality guru or another (Deming, Juran, Crosby, Berwick, Batalden, and others), the underlying concepts are similar. Quality improvement processes (as an aggregate) emphasize the total organization's integrated improvement, focusing on processes and interdepartmental involvement as well as what the consumer wants in terms of value, effectiveness, and efficiency. Continual training and education as well as committed leadership are fundamental.

- Find out if your organization has adopted the concepts of total quality management (TQM). If it has, you'll find that your leaders, from the board of directors on down, are committed to CQI (continuous quality improvement) activities, particularly in financial resource allocation, communications, and in supporting education and personnel improvement.

- Begin to plan your department's involvement according to your facility's global quality improvement initiative. You, in working with your staff and with other interfacing disciplines, will have to think about some of the following:

  ☐ Identify key procedures, functions, or services performed in your department (assessment).

  ☐ Review integral systems and processes occurring across departmental lines.

  ☐ Determine the priorities that need monitoring.

  ☐ Decide how you will know whether the important aspects are occurring correctly.

  ☐ Identify means of calling your attention to the need to evaluate. (You may have heard the Joint Commission call this identifying the methods by which you'll trigger evaluation of key indicators.)

☐ Collect information and evaluate it (more assessment data).

☐ With the team, decide how to improve the situation. (As nurses, we are now planning our interventions.)

☐ Intervene. (Do you see how cleverly the nursing process fits in here?)

☐ Evaluate the effectiveness, and communicate how well your interventions have worked. (Aha! We're now ready to assess, plan, intervene, and evaluate *again*.)

• Recognize that acronyms that seemed strange and new are really comfortable, well-worn processes, fitting with nursing's time-honored ability to provide "continually improving" quality of patient care. Now we can count on the support of health care organization executives as well as collaboration with our colleagues from other disciplines!

> *Quality, finally on the minds of all Americans, has quickly become the province of technofreaks. Every aspect of it is measured and boiled down to its quantitative essence. (That's not all bad, because (1) it puts quality solidly on the agenda, given our strong "what gets measured gets done" bias; and (2) seat-of-the-pants approaches have failed us too often in the past.) . . . My definition of quality is "I know it when I see it."*
>
> TOM PETERS

REFERENCES

O'Leary, D. O. (1991, March/April). Agenda for change initiatives: Setting the record straight. *Joint Commission Perspectives*, 1–4.

Roberts, J. & Schyve, P. (1990, May). From QA to QI: The views and roles of the Joint Commission. *The Quality Letter for Healthcare Leaders*, 9–12.

Roberts, J. S., Coale, J., & Redman, R. (1987). A history of the Joint Commission on Accreditation of Hospitals. *Journal of the American Medical Association*, *258* (7), 936–940.

Chapter 16

How Can I Thrive Instead of Barely Survive?

All we do as nurse managers is give, give, give! I was naive enough to think I could handle a demanding job with ease, plus be a part of a family, community, and do such things as water the plants and get the car oil changed as well! Well, I've had it! Something has got to give instead of me!

IF THE FACT that the dog threw up on the carpet was the last straw, it's time to stop and take stock of what's going on with the inner you. You need a break and some space for renewal. It's time to find ways to care for yourself.

Many people rely on your ability to think clearly and to be present and engaged with them individually. When you find you aren't coping effectively, it's not only damaging to you personally, but also to your department and those you serve. (The last sentence was written specifically for those of you who don't believe that it's OK for you to take care of yourself because *you* are valuable. Because we know you'll have every excuse in the world for not reading this section, we thought we'd appeal to your codependent tendencies and point out that your own state of well-being affects those you manage and want to care for.)

We also want you to know we've been at that horrid moment of exhaustion and fury, when all resources have been spent and then some. We understand the pressures, anxieties, and extreme frustration inherent in the important work we do each day while trying to live "normal" lives outside of the health care facility. And still, we've remained in health care management for decades. Keep the faith that you will be able to cope and that there will be joys to supersede the pain. We're throwing you some well-worn lifelines in the next few pages. Grab them and keep yourself afloat!

> *Exit according to rule, first leg and then head. Remove high heels and synthetic stockings before evacuation; open the door, take out the recovery line and throw it away.*

> RUMANIAN NATIONAL AIRLINES
> EMERGENCY INSTRUCTIONS

Q #70 How can I manage to cope with all this stress?

A As nurses, we teach our patients about stress reduction, about caring for themselves. Why is it so difficult for us to implement the same techniques ourselves? Think about what is preventing you from caring for yourself. If you find you are depressed or are suffering from feelings of low self-esteem, you may wish to consult with a therapist. If you don't usually understand your own body's clues to being "overheated" unless there's a boil-over (often displayed as illness or nasty behavior), perhaps you haven't taken enough time to think about your own methods of dealing with stress. A pervasive feeling of balance and peace in one's life is difficult to achieve, but implementing the following ideas have helped us to be somewhat human.

• Always be in tune with your goals and how you want to prioritize your life. What do *you* want to accomplish in life? What do you want to be remembered for when you're gone? What things are the most important to you? Does family come before work or after? What about your spiritual life? Does your bowling league and recreation come before keeping your house together? There are no wrong answers. Your responses depend on what you value in life.

- Often, feelings of stress come up when the time you are spending on one area of your life is out of equilibrium. Decide how you can readjust the balance.

- Decide what else is making you feel more stressed right now. What issues are the most pressing? As you develop action plans for resolving each one, you'll feel more relaxed. Another hint regarding each stressor: Ask yourself, "In 100 years, will this issue have any impact on the future of humankind? How important is this in the scope of the world?"

- Make an inventory of your health habits. Are you eating nutritiously? Have you kept yourself free of undue influence of drugs (including alcohol and caffeine)? Do you make sure you get aerobic exercise? We can't stress enough the positive stress reduction from exercise. This technique has saved us from inpatient psychiatric treatment more than once!

- What do you do to relax? What helps you feel more calm? Often, listening to music, chatting with good friends, taking a walk, reading a book will be useful stress reducers. Watching a video, whether you like drama to put your problem in perspective or comedy to induce cleansing laughter, helps us relax.

- Don't be afraid to ask for help, whether from a professional counselor or from a trusted friend. Just talking about worries and stress often helps reduce it.

- Take regular vacations and breaks from work. Short breaks such as long weekends, if spent doing things we like instead of overdoing on home projects, lift our spirits. Getting away for a continuing education day (taking in information instead of giving) is rejuvenating. Longer vacations are a must! We recommend at least one vacation per year that is at least two weeks long.

- Treat yourself now and then. Perhaps a treat to you is a day hunting or fishing in the wilderness; perhaps it is a new shirt or lab coat, maybe a long bath or a massage, a new hairstyle, a long distance phone call to an old friend, or a good meal in your favorite restaurant. Revel in the fact that you are alive and can enjoy the fine things in life.

- If you are still having trouble taking good care of yourself, make a list of your good qualities and remember your inherent value to yourself and to those for whom you care.

- Spend time laughing at the ridiculous things in life. If you truly look at our predicaments from the perspective of a comic, they're often quite hilarious. Some of your stressors may be the most funny. (That staff member who is attempting to pressure you out of your job by manipulative techniques is really quite entertaining if you see her antics as a spider attempting to weave a web of deceit, only to be caught in it herself!)

- Take a few deep breaths. Breathe, and close your eyes, locate yourself in a place that you love to be . . . perhaps lying on the beach with the warm sun on your skin, the sound of the waves lapping on the beach, native music, suntan oil and fragrant gardenia wafting on the breeze . . . perhaps in a mountain cabin with a sweet bird song waking you from a restful sleep, the smell of pine trees and blueberry pancakes in the air, as you snuggle under a down quilt for a few more moments of rest. Take some time each day to go to your favorite places and transport yourself out of your stressful environment, especially during those moments when you're aware of your own body signaling increasing stress.

- If you are still awake, and none of these life lines seem strong enough to pull you out of the sea of stress, keep treading water . . . and move on to the next question!

If I'd known I was gonna live this long [100 years], I'd have taken better care of myself.

EUBIE BLAKE

Q #71 What does codependence have to do with coping? (Or: If I'm a codependent nurse, can I appear on Oprah or Donahue?)

A Oh oh! As much as we'd love to avoid any more negative labels for nurses, we have seen so much evidence of codependent behaviors in nursing that it needs to be mentioned in a book for nurse managers. Not only may some of your staff members exhibit codependent behaviors, management can be a real setup for falling into the trap of feeling bad about ourselves and feeling responsible for absolutely *everything!*

Due to popular psychology, many people on talk shows have been tearfully admitting to being "codependent" because they are adult children of alcoholics or were assigned the caretaker responsibility role in their family of origin. As much as we'd like to avoid stereotyping, it's a good idea for us to recognize the potential difficulty we may have as nurses in clearly delineating our boundaries in relation to others. For example, we've seen managers who make scores of phone calls, pleading for help to cover for yet another crisis of a staff member, without dealing with the root cause of the absenteeism. We've heard managers who tolerate abusive behavior on the part of staff or other professionals, probably because they are convinced they aren't completely perfect (or worthy) and they think they should be. We've watched nurses who are extremely needy and totally dependent on the support of others, as well as those supernurses who are beyond independent and act invulnerable. We've witnessed behavior that hides anger and shame behind arrogance or "people pleasing" behavior. Dealing with these issues takes more than a two page recipe, and for some may require private therapy, but there are some strategies you can use to avoid behavior that does not support nurses' value, maturity, and accountability.

- Accept yourself the way you are. We are all in a growth curve, but learn to like yourself and respect your unique qualities and worth. Certainly you do as much for your patients.

- Be clear about your boundaries and your responsibilities. You cannot control every move of all your staff members. You are accountable to deal effectively with what does happen, but you can't stop things from going wrong. Just as nurses may become too deeply involved with patients and lose their objectivity, you too may lose your ability to problem solve well if you "become" your unit.

- Be clear about the accountability you expect from your staff. Don't take on duties that aren't yours. Don't "overparent" your staff and stop them from mature behavior. In an effort to feel better about themselves and "be liked," some managers do their staff's work. This will not foster respect for you or your role.

- Respect your strengths and those of your staff members. Expect them to respect yours and be as forgiving of your shortcomings as you are of theirs. (All of you are trying to improve, right?)

- Promote collegial relationships among your staff members and other professionals. Understanding of each other's roles and responsibilities and respect for each individual's unique contributions are essential steps.

- Whatever spirituality or religion you or your staff may practice, it is especially helpful to have some recognition of life beyond our present world when you are dealing daily with life and death. Being in tune with the eternal or spiritual life force helps people understand their inherent value, forgive themselves and others, and get on with life. In our experience, most religious beliefs encourage people to help, support, and care for themselves and each other, not based on merit, but based on intrinsic value. (Do not send in your contributions to our television ministry at this time! We are offering these thoughts to put in perspective the need for valuing yourself and others and avoiding the self-defeating relationships of codependency.)

- Learn to say "No" to duties that aren't rightfully yours.

- Have you grabbed any of these lifelines? If none of these seem to help, read on. . . .

> *The greatest danger, that of losing oneself, may pass as quietly as if it were nothing: every other loss, that of an arm, a leg, five dollars, is sure to be noticed.*
>
> SOREN KIERKEGAARD

Q #72 I sometimes find myself or my staff laughing when I'm sure we shouldn't be. Is this sick behavior?

A Saving patients' lives is serious work. Helping families grow toward optimal holistic health is serious work. We are very serious folks, we nurses. But tell me, just how serious is it when:

☐ a patient coughs so hard that sputum sticks all over the wall? (Darlene thinks the glob looks like a bedbug, Lyle thinks it looks like more like a tent caterpillar: who failed the Rorschach test?)

☐ Carrie, the charge nurse, shows up for work in two different duty shoes because she dressed in the dark? (It would catch on as a fad except for the difficulty walking with two different size heels!)

- [ ] a patient "codes" in the tubroom and the resident thinks it's OK to use the defibrillator despite the fact that everyone is now standing in water? (This gives a whole new personal meaning to the words shock, being in charge, keeping current, and sharing power!)

- [ ] a pressure bag for an arterial line is pumped up, the sterile solution bursts and is airborne, wildly spraying the room as it spins like a top, spurting nurses and physicians alike, circling the room with a life of its own? (Some vendors forgo full disclosure when it comes to the poltergeists in their intravenous solutions!)

This has been a bit of a psychological test: If you are laughing (or even smiling weakly) now, we think you are quite normal and sane. If you are disgusted that anyone could laugh at the above, we suggest that you may be taking your work a bit too seriously, and may have more trouble relieving anxieties and stress. Although pneumonia, the dress code, resuscitation, and equipment failure are serious issues, those of us who must confront daily the grave realities of life, disease, and death must be able to see the amusing, the funny, the hilarious in the human condition. (No pun intended for those of you who are truly out of control!)

- Hire people who like to laugh and enjoy life. Telling a couple of jokes or showing a related cartoon and listening to the response in the interview may reflect the applicant's ability to appreciate the ridiculous in life.

- Recognize that "gallows humor" or some of the more disgusting topics for laughter are often coping mechanisms for health care professionals. Although talking about these topics is unseemly and unprofessional outside of work or where the public may hear, it's best not to discourage this type of humor, as long it is not hurtful or disrespectful of individuals or groups.

- Encourage use of cartoons, jokes, and fun. Many units keep cartoons or humorous books and articles and videotapes in a certain area for nurses, other professionals, patients, and families. Humor has been proven to encourage healing as well as relaxation.

- Be a participant in the playtime of the group. The business world is beginning to wake up to the notion that the team that plays together stays together. Many organizations encourage onsite recreation such as miniature golf or billiards. Team sports such as hospital bowling or softball groups are common. For those who avoid athletics, a theatre critic group or gourmet club is fun.

- Use a climate of humor as a motivator and to help encourage the right brain, stimulating creativity. (Workers who feel relaxed and are free to have fun will be effective!) Modern workers expect work to be enjoyable as well as intellectually stimulating. (These reasons are given for those of you who need concrete management justification for allowing playfulness and fun in your work environment.)

- Make work fun by bringing food (always one of our favorites!), sharing a videotape library (adult video exchange may not be condoned however), having theme days, or celebrating all sorts of holidays. (Ever heard of Hug Your Computer Day? It's one our kids made up in hopes of getting gifts!) Have competition for the best fun idea. (Free coffee break for a week is motivating!) One of our favorites is charades at a staff meeting. (Name the disease is fun.)

- Learn to enjoy your work. Life is short. We can either suffer and groan and "earn" our eternal rest by the pain we endure, or we can choose to enjoy the people and circumstances we've been dealt. Somehow we think that the eternal life force must have a great sense of humor (think of some of the people you've known!), and certainly expects us to enjoy the world and each other.

Laughter is internal jogging.

NORMAN COUSINS

SUGGESTED READING

Garland, R. (1991). *Making work fun: Doing business with a sense of humor.* San Diego, CA: Shamrock Press.

Snow, C. & Willard, D. (1989). *I'm dying to take care of you: Nurses and codependence breaking the cycles.* Redmond, WA: Professional Counselor Books.

List of Sources

p. xiv   "I can tell . . ."
         Source: Copyright © 1990 by Steve Wall and Harvey Arden from the book *Wisdom Keepers*, Beyond Words Publishing, Inc., Hillsboro, Oregon.

p. 1   "We all live . . ."
         Source: Reprinted by permission of Running Press from *Quotable Women*, © 1989.

p. 4   "Don't be afraid . . ."
         Source: From Life 101: Everything We Wish We Had Learned About Life in School, But Didn't by John Roger and Peter McWilliams, published by Prelude Press, 8159 Santa Monica Boulevard, Los Angeles, California 90046, 1-800-LIFE-101, 170

p. 6   "I would not . . ."
         Source: Max DePree, *Leadership is an Art* (New York: Bantam Doubleday Dell, 1989), 22.

p. 10   "Avoiding danger is . . ."
         Source: Jennifer James, *Thinking in the Future Tense* (New York: Simon & Schuster, in press).

p. 12   "The final test . . ."
         Source: Walter Lippman

p. 16   "Good management without . . ."
         Source: Warren Bennis and Burt Nanus, *Leaders: The Strategies for Taking Charge* (New York: Harper & Row, 1985), 21.

p. 19   "Nursing's values—commitment . . ."
         Source: Leah Curtin, *Nursing Management* (West Dundee, IL: S-N Publications, 1989), 8.

p. 22   "Let whoever is . . ."
         Source: Beth T. Ulrich, *Leadership and Management According to Florence Nightingale* (East Norwalk, CT: Appleton & Lange, 1992), 38.

p. 24   "The growing American . . ."
         Source: Rhoda Thomas Tripp, *The International Thesaurus of Quotations* (New York: Harper & Row, 1970), 34.20.

p. 28   "Go put your . . ."
         Source: Anthony Robbins, *Awaken the Giant Within* (Dallas, TX: Dupree Miller Associates, 1991), 473.

p. 29   "Relationships are like . . ."
         Source: J.D. Zahniser, *And Then She Said: Quotations by Women for Every Occasion* (St. Paul, MN: Caillech Press, 1990), 46.

p. 31   "The firmest friendships . . ."
         Source: Rhoda Thomas Tripp, *The International Thesaurus of Quotations* (New York: Harper & Row, 1970), 363.31.

p. 34   "Always communicate unto . . ."
         Source: Dan Zadra, *Insights on Teamwork* (Woodinville, WA: Compendium, Inc., 1992).

p. 36   "Don't compromise yourself . . ."
         Source: Reprinted by permission of Running Press from *Quotable Women,* © 1989.

p. 38   "Be nice, feel . . ."
         Source: Walter B. Wriston

p. 41   "And that's the . . ."
         Source: From *Life 101: Everything We Wish We Had Learned About Life in School, But Didn't* by John

Roger and Peter McWilliams, published by Prelude Press, 8159 Santa Monica Boulevard, Los Angeles, California 90046, 1-800-LIFE-101, 104.

p. 44   "One only receives . . ."
Source: (Note: no author), *Each Day a New Beginning* (Center City, MN: Hazelden Foundation, 1990).

p. 47   "The world is . . ."
Source: Laurence J. Peter, *Peter's Quotations: Ideas for Our Time* (New York: William Morrow & Co., 1979), 513.

p. 49   "Never doubt that . . ."
Source: Dan Zadra, *Expect Success* (Woodinville, WA: Compendium, Inc.).

p. 52   "Let us train . . ."
Source: Laurence J. Peter, *Peter's Quotations: Ideas for Our Time* (New York: William Morrow & Co., 1979), 274.

p. 54   "Those who trust . . ."
Source: J.D. Zahniser, *And Then She Said: Quotations by Women for Every Occasion* (St. Paul, MN: Caillech Press, 1990), 47.

p. 57   "I can easier . . ."
Source: *The Oxford Dictionary of Quotations*, Third Edition (Oxford: Oxford University Press, 1979), 465.

p. 60   "Every family, every . . ."
Source: Max DePree, *Leadership is an Art* (New York: Bantam Doubleday Dell, 1989), 82.

p. 63   "The great leader . . ."
Source: Dan Zadra, *Teamwork Quotation* (Woodinville, WA: Compendium, Inc.).

p. 67   "Diversity: The art . . ."
         Source: Dan Zadra, *Teamwork Quotation* (Woodinville, WA: Compendium, Inc.).

p. 69   "Dobkins, I just . . ."
         Source: Fred Metcalf, *The Penguin Dictionary of Modern Humorous Quotations* (London: Penguin Books Ltd., 1988), 6.

p. 71   "Oh heavens, how . . ."
         Source: Tony Augarde, *The Oxford Dictionary of Modern Quotations* (Oxford: Oxford University Press, 1991), 165.15.

p. 74   "Good and evil . . ."
         Source: Anthony Robbins, *Awaken the Giant Within* (Dallas, TX: Dupree Miller Associates, 1991), 141.

p. 77   "Only children and . . ."
         Source: Lawrence C. Bassett and Norman Metzger, *Achieving Excellence: A Prescription for Health Care Managers* (Gaithersburg, MD: Aspen Publishers, Inc., 1986), 76.

p. 80   "Powerlessness corrupts. Absolute . . ."
         Source: Tom Peters, *Thriving on Chaos* (New York: St. Martins Press, 1988), 343.

p. 83   "One man may . . ."
         Source: Rhoda Thomas Tripp, *The International Thesaurus of Quotations* (New York: Harper & Row, 1970), 187.4.

p. 85   "Clapping with the . . ."
         Source: Rhoda Thomas Tripp, *The International Thesaurus of Quotations* (New York: Harper & Row, 1970), 187.3.

p. 88   "Irate, upset people . . ."
         Source: Frank C. Bucaro

p. 91   "Real nurses don't . . ."
         Source: Leah Curtin, *Nursing Management* (West Dundee, IL: S-N Publications, 1992).

p. 93   "To create an . . ."
         Source: Rhoda Thomas Tripp, *The International The-
                  saurus of Quotations* (New York: Harper &
                  Row, 1970), 392.6.

p. 95   "He has occasional . . ."
         Source: Tony Augarde, *The Oxford Dictionary of Quota-
                  tions* (Oxford: Oxford University Press, 1971),
                  511.

p. 97   "Courage is the . . ."
         Source: Amelia Earhart

p. 99   "You can't teach . . ."
         Source: Anonymous

p. 102   "To keep a . . ."
         Source: Mother Teresa

p. 104   "Things could be . . ."
         Source: Leah Curtin, *Nursing Management* (West
                  Dundee, IL: S-N Publications, 1993).

p. 107   "Relationships. That's all . . ."
         Source: J.D. Zahniser, *And Then She Said: Quotations by
                  Women for Every Occasion* (St. Paul, MN:
                  Caillech Press, 1990), 46.

p. 110   "A powerful agent . . ."
         Source: Anthony Robbins, *Awaken the Giant Within*
                  (Dallas, TX: Dupree Miller Associates, 1991),
                  200.

p. 112   "One can never . . ."
         Source: Ann Morrow Lindbergh

p. 114   "If only we'd . . ."
         Source: Edith Wharton

p. 117   "To achieve, you . . ."
         Source: Anne Wilson Schaef, *Meditations for Women
                  Who Do Too Much* (New York: Harper & Row,
                  1990), January 17.

p. 120   "Oh Great Spirit . . ."
         Source: Cherokee prayer

p. 122   "I mar the . . ."
          Source: Beth T. Ulrich, *Leadership and Management According to Florence Nightingale* (East Norwalk: CT: Appleton & Lange, 1992), 109.

p. 125   "There is never . . ."
          Source: Robert Byrne, *The Third, and Possibly the Best, 637 Things Anybody Ever Said* (New York: Macmillan, 1986), 210.

p. 127   "The length of . . ."
          Source: Rhoda Thomas Tripp, *The International Thesaurus of Quotations* (New York: Harper & Row, 1970), 230.4.

p. 131   "Tell me and . . ."
          Source: Chinese proverb

p. 133   "Man is what . . ."
          Source: Laurence J. Peter, *Peter's Quotations: Ideas for Our Time* (New York: William Morrow & Co., 1979), 39.

p. 136   "Decide what you . . ."
          Source: From *Life 101: Everything We Wish We Had Learned About Life in School, But Didn't* by John Roger and Peter McWilliams, published by Prelude Press, 8159 Santa Monica Boulevard, Los Angeles, California 90046, 1-800-LIFE-101, 208.

p. 137   "If you have . . ."
          Source: Anne Wilson Schaef, *Meditations for Women Who Do Too Much* (New York: Harper & Row, 1990), December 19.

p. 141   "Criticism is like . . ."
          Source: Rhoda Thomas Tripp, *The International Thesaurus of Quotations* (New York: Harper & Row, 1970), 204.11.

p. 143   "Before you give . . ."
          Source: Anonymous

p. 145   "Count not him . . ."
         Source: Rhoda Thomas Tripp, *The International The-
                   saurus of Quotations* (New York: Harper &
                   Row, 1970), 392.12.
p. 148   "Make it so."
         Source: "Star Trek, The Next Generation"
p. 150   "Good judgment comes . . ."
         Source: Barry LePatner
p. 154   "And the trouble . . ."
         Source: Reprinted by permission of Running Press
                   from *Quotable Women,* © 1989.
p. 155   "Life is either . . ."
         Source: Rhoda Thomas Tripp, *The International The-
                   saurus of Quotations* (New York: Harper &
                   Row, 1970), 16.4.
p. 159   "When the decision . . ."
         Source: Tony Augarde, *The Oxford Dictionary of Mod-
                   ern Quotations* (Oxford: Oxford University
                   Press, 1991), 218.13.
p. 161   "Conflict is the . . ."
         Source: North Dakota farmer
p. 164   "You cannot shake . . ."
         Source: J.D. Zahniser, *And Then She Said: Quotations by
                   Women for Every Occasion* (St. Paul, MN:
                   Caillech Press, 1990), 35.
p. 165   "Everywhere one sees . . ."
         Source: John Pekkanen, *Doctors Talk About Themselves*
                   (New York: Bantam Doubleday Dell, 1990),
                   131.
p. 169   "We have forty . . ."
         Source: Dan Zadra, *Insights on Service* (Woodinville,
                   WA: Compendium, Inc., 1992).
p. 172   "Almost means not . . ."
         Source: Dan Zadra, *Insights on Service* (Woodinville,
                   WA: Compendium, Inc., 1992).

p. 175   "To make the . . ."
          Source: John Pekkanen, *Doctors Talk About Themselves*
          (New York: Bantam Doubleday Dell, 1990).
p. 177   "Why is there . . ."
          Source: Anonymous
p. 180   "Money isn't everything . . ."
          Source: Fred Metcalf, *The Penguin Dictionary of Modern
          Humorous Quotations* (London: Penguin Books
          Ltd., 1988), 167.
p. 183   "Economists are people . . ."
          Source: Robert Byrne, *The Third, and Possibly the Best,
          637 Things Anybody Ever Said* (New York:
          Macmillan, 1986), 203.
p. 185   "There was a . . ."
          Source: Rhoda Thomas Tripp, *The International The-
          saurus of Quotations* (New York: Harper &
          Row, 1970), 596.57.
p. 187   "I have never . . ."
          Source: J.D. Zahniser, *And Then She Said: Quotations by
          Women for Every Occasion* (St. Paul, MN:
          Caillech Press, 1990), 25.
p. 190   "Reality is something . . ."
          Source: Reprinted by permission of Running Press
          from *Quotable Women,* © 1989.
p. 194   "Nurses must recognize . . ."
          Source: Tim Porter-O'Grady, *Reorganization of Nursing
          Practice: Creating the Corporate Venture*
          (Gaithersburg, MD: Aspen Publishers, Inc.,
          1990), 67.
p. 198   "I never did . . ."
          Source: Thomas Edison
p. 199   "We are all . . ."
          Source: Margaret Collier Graham
p. 202   "Bad administration, to . . ."
          Source: Rhoda Thomas Tripp, *The International The-*

saurus of Quotations (New York: Harper & Row, 1970), 13.2.

p. 204 "For is it . . ."
Source: Madame Chiang Kai-shek

p. 207 "The feeble tremble . . ."
Source: J.D. Zahniser, *And Then She Said: Quotations by Women for Every Occasion* (St. Paul, MN: Caillech Press, 1990), 42.

p. 210 "Never doubt that . . ."
Source: Dan Zadra, *Expect Success* (Woodinville: WA, Compendium, Inc.).

p. 211 "Confusion is a . . ."
Source: Rhoda Thomas Tripp, *The International Thesaurus of Quotations* (New York: Harper & Row, 1970), 255.3.

p. 214 "Robin: Batgirl! What . . ."
Source: From *Life 101: Everything We Wish We Had Learned About Life in School, But Didn't* by John Roger and Peter McWilliams, published by Prelude Press, 8159 Santa Monica Boulevard, Los Angeles, California 90046, 1-800-LIFE-101, 84.

p. 216 "Quality, finally on . . ."
Source: Tom Peters, *Liberation Management: Necessary Disorganization for the Nanosecond Nineties* (New York: Alfred A. Knopf, 1992), 677.

p. 220 "Exit according to . . ."
Source: John Roger and Peter McWilliams, *Life 101* (Los Angeles: Prelude Press, 1990), 82.

p. 223 "If I'd known . . ."
Source: Tony Augarde, *The Oxford Dictionary of Modern Quotations* (Oxford: Oxford University Press, 1991), 34.22.

p. 225   "The greatest danger . . ."
         Source: Candace Snow and David Willard, *I'm Dying
                   to Take Care of You* (Redmond, WA: Profes-
                   sional Counselor Books, 1989), 113.
p. 228   "Laughter is internal . . ."
         Source: From *Life 101: Everything We Wish We Had
                   Learned About Life in School, But Didn't* by John
                   Roger and Peter McWilliams, published by
                   Prelude Press, 8159 Santa Monica Boulevard,
                   Los Angeles, California 90046, 1-800-LIFE-
                   101, 134.

Index

About the Authors

Ruth Hansten and Marilynn Washburn are accomplished national consultants, speakers, and seminar leaders, offering a unique team approach, blending the inspirational with the practical, and humor with skill development, drawing from their years of experience in staff, middle manager, and executive positions in hospitals and other health care settings. You'll see their work widely published in nursing and management journals. Their first book, *I Light the Lamp*, is a motivational book for and by nurses, offering quotes, poems, and observations about the issues most central to the nursing profession, published in 1990 by Applied Therapeutics in Vancouver, Washington. Although nursing administration continues to be their primary focus, their comprehensive experience in consulting brings a unique approach from a multidisciplinary perspective.

For additional information or comments, contact:

Hansten and Washburn
6651 NE Baker Hill Road
Bainbridge Island, WA 98110
Telephone: 206-842-0912 or 206-842-1189
FAX: 206-842-9921

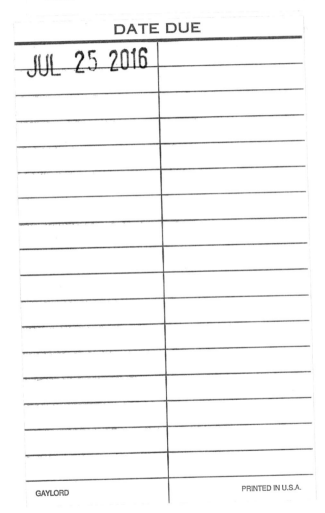

DATE DUE

JUL 25 2016

GAYLORD

PRINTED IN U.S.A.